Double Your Energy
With Half The Effort

Double Your Energy
With Half The Effort

by Judi and Shari Zucker
"The Double-Energy Twins"

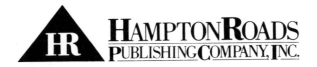
HAMPTON ROADS
PUBLISHING COMPANY, INC.

For information, write:

Hampton Roads Publishing Co., Inc.
891 Norfolk Square
Norfolk, VA 23502

Or call: 804-459-2453
    FAX: 804-455-8907

If this book is unavailable from your local bookseller, it may be obtained directly from the publisher.
Call toll-free 1-800-766-8009 (orders only).

ISBN 1-878901-18-4

10 9 8 7 6 5 4 3 2 1

Printed in the United States of America

Acknowledgements

We wish to thank our dear friends Samantha Keeping, Cristina Miles Gavin, and Kim King Fernandez for reading the manuscript multiple times and for helping us test recipes. We are also grateful to Mary Ann Painter, R.D., for her time and suggestions. Margaret Koike, a talented free-lance writer and editor assisted us in our research and in revising our original manusript, and we are very appreciative.

Special thanks to our mother, Devra Z. Hill, for her nutritional advice, love, and support. Thanks Dad (Irwin Zucker), for believing in us and promoting us like no other public relations man would! Thank you Lori Z (our sister) for your enthusiasm.

From Shari: Thank you Daniel B. Kilstofte for always encouraging me, and for being such a fabulous husband, father, and friend. Thank you Maxwell and Miles (my twin sons) for giving me a reason to keep on cooking.

Dedication

We dedicate this book to our inspirational and kind grandmother, Nanya (Giovanna Zaira Hill).

Foreword

Double Your Energy . . .
and Double Your Fun, Too

I first met Judi and Shari, the "Double-Energy Twins," back in 1979. They were fresh out of high school and riding high on the success of their first book, *How to Survive Snack Attacks . . . Naturally.* What impressed me most about the twins was their creativity and vitality—qualities that have matured with them during the last ten years. Since I first met them, Judi and Shari have also developed their expertise in cooking techniques and their firm grasp of nutritional principles.

They have now created an eating program that will appeal to and benefit practically everyone. Indeed, *Double Your Energy With Half The Effort* describes not just a sound, sensible nutritional program, but a whole way of enriching and enjoying life.

Certainly the twins exemplify this exhilarating, Santa Barbara lifestyle. They live it—and they happily share it with you in this invaluable collection of nutritional tips and recipes geared for people of all ages.

Judi and Shari don't believe in complicated cooking techniques or impossible-to-find ingredients. They make their recipes simple to cook and and delicious to eat. Their Santa Barbara lifestyle diet includes no gimmicks; it simply encourages a pure, natural way of enjoying fresh, whole foods that will promote good health and high energy—and even save you time in the kitchen.

How lucky we are that Judi and Shari are willing to show us how, with little effort, we can double our energy—and even double our joy in being alive.

Earl Mindell, Ph.D.
Author of *Unsafe at Any Meal,*
The Pill Bible, and *The Vitamin Bible*
Beverly Hills, California

Contents

Contents
(continued)

Introduction
How We Arrived

... in Santa Barbara, an oasis for the health-conscious, is a simple story to tell. We came to the University of California at Santa Barbara to study nutrition and physical education, and the area's natural beauty and invigorating climate persuaded us to stay. How we arrived at an easy-to-follow diet that reflects our city's energetic lifestyle—yet will benefit almost everyone everywhere—makes for a lengthier tale.

We became vegetarians (specifically, *lacto-ovovegetarians*, a label we'll explain in Chapter One) at the age of thirteen, when an art teacher convinced us that a meatless diet could increase our energy and improve our performance in track and field. Unfortunately, we also remained "junkatarians," aficionados of processed foods that were full of salt, white sugar, bleached white flour, potentially damaging additives, and too much fat.

But by the time we got to Santa Barbara, we had weaned ourselves from such body-damaging foods and had become proficient cooks—and voracious eaters—of whole, unprocessed, "real" foods. In fact, we had already published our first book, *How to Survive Snack Attacks ... Naturally* (1979), and we were developing plans for our next health-oriented cookbook, *How to Eat without Meat ... Naturally* (1981). Plus we had become addicted to regular aerobic exercise, which conditioned our hearts and lungs and made our energy levels soar.

We found in Santa Barbara many kindred spirits, for this small, resort city beckons those who love outdoor sports as well as freshly grown produce. Sandwiched between the Pacific Ocean and the Santa Ynez mountains on the central California coast, Santa Barbara is home to artists, writers, athletes, scholars, media celebrities, distinguished chefs, and an amazing array of health care practitioners who find the area naturally energizing.

As residents of this health-oriented town, we began to notice that most folks hereabouts are too busy to spend much time in the kitchen. Like you, they work or chase children around, and then spend evenings and weekends enjoying sports, outings, or cultural events. Yet somehow many manage to eat nutritiously, even though they may not eat the right foods at optimal times of day.

So we decided it was time to put our knowledge of nutrition

i

and exercise to work: we refined our favorite, original recipes to complement the active Santa Barbara lifestyle, and then began to spread the good word that *eating for added energy does not require a lot of time, effort, or money*. Our diet is unique in its simplicity—and in its freedom from gimmicks. Many of our easy-to-make, nutritionally balanced recipes can stand alone or serve as the heart of a meal.

We also began to tell people everywhere—including our educated Santa Barbara friends—about a daily meal pattern that can make a tremendous difference in helping one lose fat, pounds, and inches and that easily keeps extra pounds from sneaking back on. In addition, it's a unique meal plan that takes into account the fact that most of us feel much too tired to fix a large meal at the end of a long day. So many people saw so much sense in this program that they convinced us to explain it on paper. You'll find our discussion of the Light-Moderate-Light eating plan in Chapter Three.

But the singularity of *Double Your Energy With Half The Effort* doesn't stop with its Light-Moderate-Light approach to eating. Unlike many weight-reducing programs, *Double Your Energy With Half The Effort* helps you *lose weight gradually and permanently* while simultaneously boosting your energy with life-enhancing natural foods. Our *Diet* is really a whole way of life, one that can mesh with your own busy life style because the economical recipes do not require much preparation time nor large numbers of unusual ingredients. Instead, the *Diet* features *contemporary, jazzy combinations of time-honored, traditional foods* and stresses **the indisputable importance of aerobic exercise.** Based on sound nutritional and medical information, *Double Your Energy With Half The Effort* will awaken your taste buds to the sensational flavors of natural foods—and allow you to **satisfy your appetite completely.** It will help you arrive at a whole new way of choosing and eating foods.

Of course, if you have particular medical needs—or if you are pregnant, breast-feeding, or planning meals for young children—you need to consult your physician, health care-giver, or registered dietician before embarking on this or any diet. We feel certain that, because our eating program reduces the risk of many diseases and is so life-supporting, most health-care providers will endorse what lies between these covers.

So take a look. This book can change your life and double your energy!

PART I

How It Works

Chapter One

Why this "Diet" Is for You

Curiosity has gotten the better of you. As your fingers page tentatively through this volume, your eyes search skeptically for pat formulas and ambiguous promises hidden somewhere in the text. You suspect that you have your hands on yet another fad diet, and you believe that our "dietetic" recipes will ask you to ingest palm fronds, sea urchins, or piles of avocados simply so that you can savor the flavors of our city.

And who ever heard of a diet that can double your energy? All the diets you've tried have only made you feel tired and hungry. Perhaps those regimens left your wallet a bit tired, too. And maybe you ended up with more weight than you had when you began the diet.

Before you put this book down, skim through the chapters and examine the recipes carefully. You'll quickly discover that we use the term "diet" in its original sense; after all, the word simply refers to whatever each of us eats every day. Like many of today's nutritionists and health-care advisors, we want to encourage a way of eating that you can follow for the *rest* of your life—not just for a week or a month.

In this book we do just that; we propose a way of eating that will do the following:

- satisfy your physical hunger as well as your psychological needs for chewy, crunchy, smooth, tangy, or sweet foods
- fulfill all your nutritional needs
- negate your need to count calories
- drastically reduce the amount of fat in your meals
- significantly lower your chances for developing cancer, heart disease, hypertension, diabetes, osteoporosis, and diverticulitis (inflammations in the intestinal tract)
- help you avoid consuming concentrated amounts of pesticides and other food contaminants
- save you time in the kitchen
- reduce your food budget
- prevent needless suffering of animals
- help conserve some of the world's energy resources
- boost your body's energy to new heights

No, we're not pitching a miracle diet. If you want to succeed at this rather relaxed eating program, you will need to choose your foods wisely, exercise moderately, and allow your body time to adjust to the changes you're instigating. However, you'll be able to eat as much as you can hold of an incredible array of whole, nutritious foods; because such foods are bulky and filling, you will have a tough time gaining additional weight, and you won't have to bother with calorie counts. You will simply need to moderate your intake of sweets and naturally fatty foods, like cheeses and nuts. Of course, such moderation will become second nature once you reeducate your taste buds to the glories of grains, legumes, fruits, and vegetables.

No doubt you'll quickly discover that the *Double Your Energy With Half the Effort* diet is exceptionally **EASY** to follow and that the foods you crave are **SIMPLE** and **QUICK** to prepare. In fact, most of the recipes in this book can stand by themselves as light or moderate meals, accompanied simply by bread, a cooked grain, or a fresh fruit or vegetable. With little effort, you can make permanent changes in your lifestyle—and save money, too. Even exercise will become an addictive activity for you, and you will enjoy more energy than you've ever had before.

What do we mean by "energy"? *Simply defined, energy is an inherent capacity for work, for vigorous activity.* The word also denotes the resources—the fuel—used to produce energy in such forms as heat, motion, and electricity. Human energy—our ability to sustain ourselves and to move—comes from the energy supplied by elements in food, water, and air. We know that you're quite familiar with the term *calorie*, but did you know that it measures energy? A calorie is not some magical expression of the weight-building capacity of foods; it is the amount of heat energy you need to raise the temperature of one gram of water one degree centigrade, and it's the term scientists use to describe the *energy value* of foods.

How does the *Double Your Energy With Half The Effort* diet supply bodies with extra energy? The answer is very straightforward: the diet revolves around complex carbohydrates, which are the essential constituents of foods that come from plants. As you'll see in the next chapter, complex carbohydrates are the nutrients that supply our systems with the best and most readily available energy. According to Harold McGee's authoritative kitchen reference titled *On Food and Cooking*, our bodies find "carbohydrates . . . the preferred energy source, the first to be tapped, and when adequately supplied, they spare both fats and proteins from being consumed."[1] Complex carbohydrates supply energy that the body can use efficiently and evenly over time, and they also come packaged with essential amino acids, the building blocks of protein, which are essential to our bodies' growth.

Because foods derived from plants are so beneficial, and because they have been the staples in so many cultures for so many centuries, we have designed our recipes and menus to be essentially **lacto-ovo-vegetarian**. In other words, the *Double Your Energy With Half The Effort* diet centers on plant foods plus dairy products and eggs, which add variety and provide necessary minerals and vitamins, including riboflavin, calcium and vitamins A, B_{12}, and D. They also supply protein that the body uses even more efficiently than the protein available in meat, fish, or poultry.

If you aren't sure whether you want to embark upon a vegetarian regime, simply try cutting back on the amount of meat you normally eat. As researchers have stated countless times in the last decade or so, Americans eat far too much animal protein, and because that protein usually comes bundled with saturated fats and potentially high levels of contaminants like pesticides and antibiotics, meat consumption probably contributes to atherosclerosis (blockage of arteries and thickening of artery walls), heart disease, cancer, and other serious illnesses. (See Chapter Two for a comprehensive look at the problems inherent in animal protein.) If you can begin to use meat simply as an accompaniment to a main dish of grains, legumes, and/or vegetables, you will soon find that your taste for animal flesh will decrease. Your palate will change, and you may find it quite easy to eliminate meats from your diet entirely.

Even if you choose to eat meat, poultry, or fish now and then, the recipes in this book will probably help you to move toward an ideal body weight, to maintain that weight, to cut down the amount of unnecessary fat tissue in your body, and maybe even to live a longer, more energetic life.

In fact, once you educate your taste buds to the lovely flavors of whole, unprocessed foods, the ingredients fundamental to our recipes will become staples in your kitchen and your diet. And because you can eat a much higher volume of these complex-carbohydrate foods than animal foods for the same number of calories, you will find that you can satisfy your appetite without worrying about calorie counts. High-carbohydrate diets like this one are naturally low in fat, and medical researchers have shown that diets which focus on decreasing fat rather than decreasing calories allow individuals to lose weight spontaneously and to maintain near-ideal weights. Plus those individuals can eat as much as they like of delicious, low-fat foods.[2]

Further, the *Double Your Energy With Half The Effort* diet proposes a way of eating that is incredibly economical for yourself and for the world. Grains, legumes, fruits, and vegetables cost so little compared to meats, and they require much less energy output to get them from the field to your table. According to Frances Moore Lappé's revolutionary book *Diet for a Small Planet;* a rancher requires sixteen pounds of grain and soybeans to produce just one pound of beef.[3] Just think how many mouths in a Third World country those sixteen pounds would feed! A meal of grain and soybeans supplies much more usable protein than you can find in one pound of meat, and these plant foods contain no saturated fat or cholesterol.

So not only will following a whole-foods diet increase your personal energy, it will preserve some of our environment's energy resources. In a sense it is a transforming diet, an eating plan that is life-preserving. As Lappé notes so eloquently in her first chapter, "what we eat is within our control, yet the act ties us to the economic, political, and ecological order of our whole planet. Even an apparently small change—consciously choosing a diet that is good both for our bodies and for the earth—can lead to a series of choices that transform our whole lives."[4]

Such a diet can transform our future, too: as you'll read in Chapter Three, medical researchers have amassed much evidence that too much fat in the diet creates a high risk of colon cancer, breast cancer, atherosclerosis, heart disease, gallstones, and other major health problems. What's more, certain fruits and vegetables, including citrus fruits, cabbage, cauliflower, broccoli, spinach, legumes, and seeds, may actually help prevent cancer by encouraging the body's production of certain enzymes.[5] As you'll discover, the recipes in *Double Your Energy With Half The Effort* focus on these life-sustaining plant foods, ones that may actually revitalize and prolong your life.

Chapter Two

Uppers and Downers:
Food and Your Energy Levels

To appreciate the simplicity of *Double Your Energy With Half The Effort*, you need at least to survey the complex chemistry of all the foods available to us. Many medical researchers and dieticians have spent lifetimes exploring the intricacies of nutrients and energy balances in humans.

Because we like to keep nutritional information intelligible, we refer to those foods which our bodies convert efficiently to usable energy *and* which supply important nutrients as "**uppers**." These are the foods at the heart of *Double Your Energy With Half The Effort*. At the other end of the food spectrum are "**downers**," energy sources that transform easily into detrimental body fat, contribute to risk for disease, or carry little nutritional value. To clarify what we mean by "uppers" and "downers," we need to discuss the chemical compounds that distinguish the three main food groups that fuel our bodies: proteins, fats, and carbohydrates. Because each serves a necessary function, we cannot label any of these energy sources as strictly an "upper" or a "downer"; each can be either, depending upon a number of criteria.

PROTEIN

Protein is essential to our bodies' ability to create tissues, to make disease-fighting antibodies, to regulate acidity and alkalinity levels, to move nutrients and oxygen in and out of cells throughout our bodies, and to help blood clot. Although protein exists in every cell of our bodies, we must replenish our protein supply daily because the human anatomy simply cannot store this invaluable fuel and because a protein deficiency can cause muscle loss. The protein our bodies need for all of the above functions comes from food protein, which consists of many different amino acids; the human body takes apart these dietary amino acids and creates new ones. However, of the 22 amino acids humans need to survive, 8 must be supplied directly from food because our bodies cannot manufacture them. These 8 *essential amino acids,* all of which must be present in our systems simultaneously in order for them to do us any good, are *isoleucine, leucine, lysine, methionine, threonine, valine, phenylalanine,* and *tryptophan.* In addition, the amino acid *histidine* is essential to children's growth.

When the essential amino acids are present together in a food, nutritionists say that the food supplies **complete protein**; in other words, one can eat that food alone and have all his or her protein needs met. All foods which come from animals (meats, eggs, and milk products—every animal-supplied food except gelatin) furnish the body with complete protein; a single plant food offers only some of the essential amino acids and therefore provides incomplete protein if one eats that food by itself.

What turns animal proteins into "downer" foods, however, is the cholesterol and fat—highly saturated, artery-damaging fat—with which those proteins come packaged. In fact, many animal proteins contain more fat than protein, and they offer the body absolutely no fiber, so one tends to eat more than one needs.

Indeed, as researchers point out repeatedly, we Americans consume far more protein—particularly animal protein—than we can ever possibly use. Only about ten to fifteen percent of the adult male's diet needs to consist of protein. Of that protein, only twenty percent needs to be complete.[1] Our bodies use protein for energy only after we burn fats and carbohydrates. Excess protein simply converts to fat, a body component few of us need to gain.[2] Plus too much protein prompts the body to lose bone-building calcium, contributes to high blood pressure, and can eventually damage the kidneys because they cannot process all the extra nitrogen that is intrinsic to protein.[3]

Furthermore, scientists have found increasing evidence that red meat and poultry, most folks' principal sources of protein, may contain dangerous, concentrated levels of contaminants, such as the pesticides applied to the grains that animals eat in such great quantities. The meat Americans eat may also harbor the antibiotics and hormones that ranchers use to prevent disease and to promote growth in livestock. Even fish, which offer humans beneficial unsaturated fat, are potential sources of food poisoning because of the toxic microorganisms the fish have consumed. Fish may also contain dangerous chemical contaminants like DDT or polychlorinated biphenyls (PCBs).

Consumption of chemicals harbored in the flesh of livestock, poultry, and fish may someday cause health problems for humans.[4]

To circumvent such problems—and to save an immense amount of money—one can acquire all the complete protein he or she needs from plant foods (preferably organically grown), which possess varying amounts and numbers of the eight essential amino acids. How? By combining different kinds of plant foods, a trick that people from many cultures have done for centuries without even understanding just what they were doing. Many cultural groups have flourished on cuisines that featured very little animal protein but large portions of grains and legumes.

Even strict vegetarians (often called *vegans*) who eat nothing other than plant foods can live quite normally if they combine the right foods. And lacto-ovovegetarians like us have no problem meeting their daily protein requirements. In fact, we don't even think about **protein complementarity,** the balancing of one food with another so that our bodies receive adequate but not excessive protein; food combining comes naturally, as it probably will to you, too.

Simply remember these basic protein combinations of "upper" foods, used often in *Double Your Energy With Half The Effort,* when planning your menus:

1. **Grains + legumes**
2. **Grains, seeds, nuts, or legumes + milk products or eggs**
3. **Seeds or nuts + legumes**

If you eat any one of these "upper" food combinations at the same meal, your body will amass all of the amino acids it needs to function properly. The bases for human diets in many countries for countless centuries, the *grains* called for above include corn, wheat, oats, buckwheat (really a seed), rice, rye, barley, sorghum, amaranth, millet, and all of grains' manifestations: breads, cereals, pastas, crackers, couscous, tortillas, dumplings, and so on. Extremely high in valuable nutrients, *legumes* (dried peas and beans) have likewise fueled the forgers of great civilizations. The legume family includes peanuts, lentils, chickpeas (garbanzo beans), black beans, various white beans, split peas, kidney beans, lima beans, pinto beans, blackeyed peas, red beans, and more. The legume food group also includes the amazing soybean; these versatile beans offer humans a nearly complete form of protein. (By the way, those concerned about the flatulence caused by the indigestible sugars in legumes can simply soak their beans overnight or for at least a few hours before cooking and then discard the soaking water. Combining beans with other foods will also reduce the problem—and you don't need to eat a lot of beans to reap their benefits.)

Seeds and *nuts*, powerhouses of protein, complement other plant foods superbly. However, these high-energy foods also contain plenty of fat (though mostly unsaturated) and calories, so enjoy them in moderation, and try to limit yourself to the dry-roasted, unsalted varieties. Technically speaking, seeds, which come from the fruits of plants and contain the embryos for the next generation of their species, include cashews, Brazil nuts, pumpkin and squash seeds, sesame seeds, and sunflower seeds. The dried fruit of trees, edible nuts include chestnuts, almonds, hazelnuts (filberts), pignoli (pine nuts), pecans, pistachios, and walnuts.

When you consider adding seeds or nuts to your meals, please note that macadamias and coconuts, two favorite snack foods, won't qualify for protein complementarity. Macadamias are seeds that contain little protein and lots of fat. In addition, coconuts are not protein-packed nuts at all; rather, they are *drupes*—fruits with hard stones at their centers, as are plums and apricots—that contain excessive amounts of saturated fat which may be more harmful to blood vessels than either butter or lard.[5]

As we mentioned earlier, *milk products* and *eggs* provide complete protein in themselves. Further, their protein power multiplies when you combine them with plant foods. However, as in the case of seeds and nuts, you need to use these foods in conjunction with others so that you won't consume too much fat or cholesterol. Go especially easy on the eggs: the yolk of a single egg, which holds all kinds of wonderful nutrients, also contains almost the maximum amount of cholesterol you should consume in a single day. More on milk products in the next section.

Combining different plant and dairy foods will no doubt come naturally and simply once you've tried it a few times. You won't need any tables or charts or figures. You've probably created complementary proteins in the past without even knowing it: think how often you've eaten pizza, macaroni and cheese, cereal with milk, peanut-butter sandwiches, bean burritos, muffins, pasta with dairy-based sauces, rice and beans, pancakes, and stir-fried veggies and nuts served with rice. The only hitch in creating complementary proteins is to avoid using too much cheese or too many eggs, ingredients that contain large amounts of saturated fat, which may negate some of the value of your otherwise nutritious meal.

FATS

Complete protein that comes from animals most often travels with large quantities of dietary fat, a substance that provides plenty of energy—at a high price. A potential "downer" food, fat contains more than twice as many calories (9) per gram as proteins (4) or carbohydrates (4), it provides our organs with few nutrients, and it poses serious health risks to those whose daily intake of fat exceeds thirty percent of their total calories. And it's easy to eat too much fat because you must eat more to feel full and because fat tastes so good to most of us.

You may be surprised to learn that you don't need to eat fat in order to manufacture the fat your body needs to survive. Body fat insulates and cushions your organs and provides oils for your hair and skin. If you are a woman, you need fat to help build prostaglandins, the chemicals that regulate your sex hormones. Nonetheless, each of us only needs to consume one tablespoon of fat per day to maintain good nutrition. Our bodies use proteins and carbohydrates to manufacture body fat for calorie storage, and our systems only need that one tablespoon of *polyunsaturated* fat from a vegetable source in order to obtain the essential chemical called *linoleic acid,* which we need to create body fat. That one tablespoon of polyunsaturated fat also helps our digestive system absorb the fat-soluble vitamins A, D, E, and K. However, our anatomies need absolutely no *saturated* fat—the kind that comes from animal foods. What do the terms *polyunsaturated* and *saturated* mean? You've probably heard the word *polyunsaturated* applied to the cooking oils you buy at your supermarket. Really, there are three kinds of dietary fats—those that contain primarily *saturated, polyunsaturated,* and *monounsaturated* fatty acids— but you may not have heard much about the last. And what is all the commotion about *cholesterol*? What does it have to do with fats and oils?

Saturated fats, the "downer" fats that pose the greatest danger to our health, occur in animal tissues and in the coconut oil, palm oil, palm-kernel oil, and cocoa butter so frequently used in candies and processed foods. For those interested in the technical side of things: These fats acquired their name because the fatty acids, composed of carbon and hydrogen atoms, that make up saturated fats have no double or triple bonds and no more room for any additional hydrogen—in other words, the molecules are completely full or "saturated." Solid at room temperature, saturated fats are easy to recognize. Butter, lard, chicken fat, and all that marbling in "high-quality" meats are saturated fats that researchers link to cancers of the colon, breast, uterus, ovaries, and other parts of the body. Plus saturated fats clog circulatory systems and cause heart disease.Cholesterol is not the same thing as saturated fat; it is a lipid molecule found in all animals, including those with little or no saturated fat, like shellfish. However, saturated fat and cholesterol often travel hand-in-hand, and saturated fat provokes your body's own cholesterol-manufacturing machine.

Humans need cholesterol to make cell membranes and certain hormones, and to form vitamin D molecules. We also need this vital substance to produce bile salts that help the intestine metabolize dietary fats. However, after the age of six months, our bodies can synthesize—in the liver, intestine, and elsewhere—all the cholesterol we need without the assistance of additional dietary cholesterol.[6] Although eating foods that contain cholesterol decreases the amount of cholesterol produced by the liver, the synthesis of cholesterol continues to some extent in other tissues.[7] In addition, some studies indicate that dietary cholesterol may not be used in the same way in which our naturally synthesized cholesterol is used; in fact, dietary cholesterol may go almost directly to the blood vessels.[8] Thus we end up with far more cholesterol in our bodies than we need. Indeed, we have difficulty getting rid of excess cholesterol that accumulates in our bodies and becomes deposited in our blood vessels. Scientists now believe that physical inactivity and emotional stress also increase the amount of cholesterol in our blood.[9]

To complicate matters further, our bodies possess what mass-media health literature calls "good" cholesterol and "bad" cholesterol. You see, cholesterol gets around in the blood by means of complex substances that are both fat (lipid) and protein. These cholesterol-carrying *lipoproteins* come in three main varieties: *high-density lipoproteins (HDLs), low-density lipoproteins (LDLs),* and *very-low-density lipoproteins (VLDLs).* In general, medical scientists refer colloquially to the HDLs as "good" because they take cholesterol away from the artery walls and transport it to the liver, where the HDLs also help to eliminate excess cholesterol. For these reasons, HDLs, which are the primary vehicles by which fats derived from plant foods travel, seem to prevent heart and artery disease. Aerobic exercise seems to increase the levels of HDL-transported cholesterol.

On the other hand, LDLs and VLDLs, low-density and very-low-density lipoproteins, arise in the liver when the diet contains lots of saturated fats, and they tend to keep cholesterol in circulation. They deliver cholesterol to cells that need it, but they fail to remove excess cholesterol from artery walls. Most of the cholesterol in our bodies travels inside LDLs and VLDLs, the notoriously "bad" kind of cholesterol carrier.

Polyunsaturated fats, which are those supplied by plant foods, travel primarily via HDLs, which reduce the amount of cholesterol in your blood and may help to lower blood pressure. These fats acquired their name ("poly" means "many") because their fatty acid molecules contain more than one double or triple bond between hydrogen and carbon clusters and can accept at least four more hydrogen atoms. Polyunsaturated fats occur as oils at room temperature, and they include soybean, safflower, sunflower, corn, linseed (which, like fish, contains valuable Omega-3 fatty acids) and cottonseed oils, as well as the fats in most nuts.

Monounsaturated fats, whose fatty acid molecules have just one double bond and can accept just two more hydrogen atoms, include olive oil, peanut oil, and the fats in avocados and cashews. Unlike polyunsaturated oils, these fats tend to thicken when refrigerated. Monounsaturated fats may be even more effective in reducing cholesterol in our blood than polyunsaturated oils.

Although monounsaturated and polyunsaturated oils qualify as "upper" foods when used sparingly, they can be problematic for our bodies if food manufacturers have *hydrogenated* them. Hydrogenation is a process by which a polyunsaturated or monounsaturated oil is made more saturated, as in the case of many margarines and vegetable shortenings. According to some studies, hydrogenated oils may allow cancer-causing chemicals easier access to certain cells.[10] Thus, if you are looking for a good margarine, check the ingredients label and choose softer rather than harder versions. Because of the problems surfacing as a result of hydrogenated fat consumption, we prefer to use completely natural fats like safflower oil, olive oil, or very small amounts of butter—even though it is saturated—when we cook. (Also, we favor just a touch of raw certified butter as an accompaniment to fresh bread. Raw certified butter contains no added salt and has not been pasteurized.)

When selecting a cooking fat, simply remember that too much of any kind of fat increases body weight, and studies are beginning to indicate that large amounts of even the unsaturated fats may contribute to the development of cancer and of gallstones. Plus, unknown to you, your body may be genetically predisposed to produce far more "bad" cholesterol than "good" cholesterol—no matter which kind of fat you eat. For these reasons, we have designed *Double Your Energy With Half The Effort*, an eating plan high in complex carbohydrates, to limit almost automatically the amount of fat you consume to 30 percent or less of your total calorie intake, a percentage recommended by the Senate Select Committee on Nutrition and Human Needs in its landmark report *Dietary Goals for the United States.*[11]

CARBOHYDRATES

Increasing your consumption of whole foods that contain complex carbohydrates and fiber will quite naturally lead to a decrease in dietary fat because complex-carbohydrate foods usually contain little fat—and no deadly saturated fat—and because such foods fill you up without filling you with calories. Contrary to popular belief, most "natural" carbohydrates are not fattening at all! They are the "upper" foods you combine to create complete, usable proteins. (See the section on proteins above.) What's more, complex carbohydrates are an incredible source of efficiently burned energy.

Complex carbohydrates are one of two major types of carbohydrate, an organic compound composed of carbon, hydrogen, and oxygen. The complex type are starches that consist of long chains of sugar molecules which our bodies break down gradually, thus releasing energy incrementally. The grains, legumes, vegetables, fruits, seeds, and nuts we discussed in the above section on complementary proteins are complex-carbohydrate foods.

The other type of carbohydrate is the **simple carbohydrate**, composed of just one or two molecules of sugar. These simple sugars include *fructose*, *glucose*, and *sucrose*, or table sugar.

Plants make both simple and complex carbohydrates during photosynthesis, the process by which water, carbon dioxide, and sunlight become chemical energy. Milk, which contains the sugar *lactose*, is the only food from an animal source that possesses a carbohydrate in any significant amount.

Once we eat any kind of carbohydrate, our bodies break it down into glucose, which circulates through the body and supplies the cells with their favorite kind of fuel. Interestingly, the brain and other tissues in the nervous system can use *only* glucose for energy; fats simply won't do.[12] Our bodies can store only about one-half a day's supply of glucose as *glycogen* in the liver and muscles, and we will begin to convert (inefficiently and sometimes dangerously) body proteinand fat into glucose if our glycogen supply runs short. If we must rely on protein or fat for our glucose, we overtax our kidneys and can cause our bodies serious harm. Humans cannot function properly without the right glucose levels; if our metabolism of the substance goes awry, we end up with diabetesor hypoglycemia. If all of the carbohydrates we eat end up as glucose, why does *Double Your Energy With Half The Effort* revolve around complex rather than simple carbohydrates? Aren't all carbohydrates the same in the end? And aren't straight sugars better sources of quick energy than are complex carbohydrates?

Sure, but therein lies the problem: the energy from simple carbohydrates is much too quickly enjoyed. Not only do the sugars in candy bars, soft drinks, or table sugar rot your teeth, they also cause a sugar "high" that is followed rapidly by a crash in blood sugar. These "downer" foods trigger excessive bursts of insulin, the hormone that regulates blood sugar levels, which rapidly takes care of *all* the sugar in the blood. A sugar low can leave you feeling a little depressed and probably even hungrier than you were before.

In addition, sugars that don't travel with starches, or complex carbohydrates, provide little in the way of nutrients. Simple carbohydrates are those "empty calories" you've heard so much about. When we use them as substitutes for other foods, simple carbohydrates may prevent us from obtaining the vitamins and minerals we need. Even honey, which is preferable to refined sugar because it contains a few trace minerals and usually tastes more potent per teaspoon than refined sugars, has minimal nutritional value. (Please note: *never* give honey to infants under one year of age. Doctors link honey with infant botulism, a food poisoning that is usually fatal.) The only sweetener with any real food value is molasses, and the darker the molasses the better. Some complex carbohydrates fit into the "empty calorie" group, too. These are the refined complex carbohydrates, which are the processed starches included in many cookies, cakes, and other desserts.

On the other hand, the complex carbohydrates found in fruits, vegetables, grains, and beans come with wide varieties of nutrients and various forms of **fiber**, the plant substances (cellulose, hemicellulose, pectin, lignin, gums, mucilage, and polysaccharides) that our human digestive enzymes cannot break down. Dietary fiber makes us feel full and keeps our digestive tract in top shape. In addition, scientific studies show that the dietary fiber in complex carbohydrates acts as a natural laxative and prevents bowel disease, heart disease, and cancers of the colon and breast. Fiber satisfies our psychological need to chew, absorbs water and makes us feel full, interferes with the body's absorption of fats, and indirectly changes the amount of glucose we absorb. Thus a fiber-rich diet may quite naturally reduce the calories, cholesterol, and saturated fats we consume.[13] Fruits, vegetables, and bran-containing whole grains are the best sources of dietary fiber.

Fiber-rich complex carbohydrates can supply our bodies with all the vitamins, minerals, protein, and fat necessary for healthy living.Investigations of traditional diets, such as those of many African and Chinese people, and scientific research suggest that up to 60 percent of our total food energy should come from complex carbohydrates.[14] In addition, complex-carbohydrate whole foods have not been associated in any way with any major disease. And because digestive enzymes break complex carbohydrates into glucose slowly, plant foods cause our blood sugar levels to stay pretty even and make energy available to us for a relatively long period of time. .And energy is what we're after!

OTHER UPPERS & DOWNERS

As you've seen in our discussion above, complex carbohydrates are the primary "upper" food fuels for our bodies. Some dietary proteins and fats also qualify, but only complex carbohydrates from "natural," unprocessed foods supply all the nutrients we need without contributing any negative factors. Another essential "upper" fuel is **water**, our bodies' most critical nutrient and lubricant. A simple combination of hydrogen and oxygen, water is the substance that composes about 60 to 70 percent of our body weight and is the main constituent of blood. Water keeps everything in our bodies moving, speeds fat metabolism, and regulates our internal temperature. For those of us on high-carbohydrate, high-fiber diets, water is especially important for keeping our digestion and elimination systems in good working order.

Unfortunately, many of us drink water that contains contaminants which may interfere with good health. Tap water may even contain suspected carcinogens, cancer-causing elements, like polychlorinated biphenyls (PCBs) and chloroform. Contamination from viruses, bacteria, pesticides, toxic heavy metals, industrial chemicals, asbestos, and simply the additives cities use to treat public water can cause serious medical problems. Some water supplies also contain excessive amounts of sodium. If you drink your water straight from the tap, be sure to have it tested periodically for contaminants. And if the water coming from your faucet ever looks cloudy, boil it for at least ten minutes before using it to cook or drink. Better yet, investigate the home filtration systems available for purchase. Check out reverse-osmosis systems, distillers, activated carbon filters, and commercially bottled waters. Each has its benefits and drawbacks, but all probably provide higher quality water than does your tap. For an informative overview of all these water options, take a look at Earl Mindell's extremely helpful book titled *Unsafe at Any Meal* (New York: Warner Books, 1987).

While we're speaking about the liquid so essential to our bodies, we should mention several beverages that many people imbibe in place of water, but which certainly qualify as "downers" for our metabolisms.

Probably the most detrimental beverage you can drink is **alcohol**, which clearly qualifies as an "empty-calorie" food because it contains plenty of simple sugars but no nutrients. People who drink alcohol in excess tend to consume little else and can eventually suffer from malnutrition and dehydration; not only does alcohol contain no vitamins or minerals, it also draws water out of brain cells and prevents your body from absorbing nutrients from other foods. Because alcohol is also a drug that alters brain functions and acts as anesthetic, its consumption is the primary cause of almost half our nation's traffic accidents each year.[15] And, as you already know, medical scientists link heavy drinking with liver disease, high blood pressure, stroke, heart disease, cancer, and fetal alcohol syndrome, the terribly sad condition affecting babies of women who drink heavily during their pregnancies. Even a few alcoholic drinks can depress one's immune system and increase one's susceptibility to infections, and alcohol can react adversely with many medications. In fact, the additives in many alcoholic beverages can cause adverse reactions all by themselves. Need we say more?

Other mind-altering "downer" beverages that need to be eliminated from a sound diet are **coffee, tea, cocoa,** and **colas.** These beverages contain *caffeine,* *theophylline* and/or *theobromine,* stimulants that affect the heart, brain, central nervous system, respiratory system, and kidneys. Like alcohol, they dehydrate rather than replenish your body's fluid supply; these stimulants stress the kidneys and act as diuretics. Although caffeine-containing beverages can speed up the rate at which you metabolize fuels, they can also increase your hunger because they stimulate the release of insulin, which clears glucose from your blood. Caffeine-containing drinks may indeed make you more mentally alert for a while, but your body will come to depend on them, and withdrawal from the beverages can result in headaches, depression, fatigue, nausea, and a number of other symptoms. Although caffeine consumption may not increase the risk for major cancers, as many once thought,[16] researchers have linked high caffeine intake with higher incidences of miscarriage among pregnant women as well as high blood pressure and elevated blood cholesterol.[17] As you see, caffeine-containing beverages can sabotage an otherwise nutritious diet and healthy lifestyle, and they can trigger the same sorts of energy crashes that sweets do.

Colas also pose another problem: like all other **soft drinks**, they leach calcium from our systems, interfere with iron absorption, dose our bodies with potentially harmful additives (like brominated vegetable oils and sodium alginate), give us quick energy fixes that end up as energy crashes, provide us with no nutritive value except almost pure calories, and bolster our craving for additional sweets. Even diet soft drinks condition us to crave sugar because the body believes it is consuming huge amounts of sugar and acts accordingly. Diet drinks prevent us from reconditioning our palate to desire fewer sweeteners, and diet beverages contain far too much sodium, another potential "downer."

While alcohol and caffeine cause the loss of valuable fluids, another chemical, **salt**, or sodium chloride, can cause excessive retention of fluids, resulting in high blood pressure and fatigue. Forty percent of the salt molecule is sodium, the mineral necessary for many of our bodies' functions—and the mineral responsible for such conditions as the hypertension mentioned above and the bloated feeling associated with premenstrual tension. Sodium occurs naturally in plenty of whole, unprocessed foods, and certain vegetables and dairy products (such as celery, spinach, beets, cheeses, and eggs) possess high levels of the mineral. But what concerns dieticians and physicians is the sodium that we add to our foods either by processing or canning them or simply by passing the salt shaker over perfectly tasty foods. (Examples of highly salted packaged or prepared foods include potato chips, pickles, ready-to-eat cereals, instant puddings, canned vegetables, commercially baked goods, and, of course, processed meats, which also contain other dangerous additives.) You will obtain more than enough sodium to regulate the fluids in your membranes if you stick to recipes in *Double Your Energy With Half The Effort*, and by weaning yourself from added salt, you can fight fatigue and appreciate the flavors of whole foods even more. Discover the unique culinary personalities of fresh or dried herbs, which make terrific, healthful alternatives to table salt, the ultimate "downer" food additive.

The final "downer" we need to mention is **tobacco**, which may be the Western world's greatest health danger. According to World Health Surveys, smoking plays a direct role in more than 500,000 American deaths yearly, including those from cancer, heart disease, respiratory disease, fire, and other accidents. The annual number of deaths caused by cigarette smoking is greater than the total number of American casualties during World War II. And these figures may be understated.[18] Furthermore, passive smoking, or the breathing of someone else's tobacco smoke, may also damage the lungs, particularly those of children. The Environmental Protection Agency has stated that passive smoke is "the most dangerous airborne carcinogen" in the U.S. The EPA estimates that between 500 and 5,000 Americans die each year because they have had to breathe someone else's cigarette smoke.[19]

For those who want to maintain good health, smoking must have no place in their lives *at all*. Not only does smoking cause fatal diseases, it interferes with the absorption of vital nutrients, and it causes a significant vitamin C deficit in the blood.

In summary, then, we recommend that you ease yourself into *Double Your Energy* diet by moving toward a healthier lifestyle:

- Avoid "downer" foods—meats (which are high in saturated fats and cholesterol), large amounts of any kind of fat, and foods with lots of sugar or salt.
- Drop all "downer" beverages—alcohol, caffeine-containing beverages, and soft drinks—from your diet.
- Eat a wide variety of "upper" foods—complex carbohydrates and low-fat or nonfat dairy products—to promote high energy.
- Drink plenty of water and juices (about eight glasses a day) to keep your body operating in high gear.

Chapter Three

Light-Moderate-Light:
A Meal Pattern that Works

Now that you have a grasp of the kinds of foods that will spur your energy, you need to think about the times of day at which you'll eat those vitalizing foods. *When* you eat is almost as important as *what* you eat. As we've said before, you'll eventually retrain your taste buds and your metabolism so that you can pretty much eat as much as you want of what we call "upper" foods. However, you will find that your body will maintain peak energy levels if you plan your meals to accommodate your body's natural rhythms—if you eat **a light breakfast, a moderate lunch,** and **a light dinner.** A meal pattern that's unique to *Double Your Energy With Half The Effort* in that it contradicts contemporary practices as well as most other diets' recommendations, this plan nonetheless reflects the traditional eating patterns of other cultures.

Delaying or omitting any meal may make you feel cranky and fatigued; hunger can even cause symptoms like headaches and dizziness. On the other hand, eating gobs of food when your body doesn't need much or eating late at night when it can't burn calories effectively can bring on bulges where you don't want them.

Amazingly, healthy bodies have an innate knowledge about when and how much to eat. Sure, certain areas of your mind often override the brain's own intuitive sense of what's right for the stomach, especially when you're feeling depressed, unhappy, or angry. But even if you're not in reasonable physical shape at the moment, you can learn how to tune in to the wisdom of your own body—how to pay attention to the signals emitted by the parts of the brain that regulate hunger and thirst. And you can become aware of your circadian rhythms. What do we mean by **circadian rhythms**? They're the biological rhythms that govern the inner workings of humans, the ones that tend to synchronize with what's going on in our environments but that don't depend on anything external to us. A chronobiologist (a scientist who studies time cycles in the natural world) named Franz Halberg first introduced the term while conducting experiments in Minneapolis in 1959; Halberg used it to describe biological rhythms that have a period of about 24 hours (*circa diem*, Latin for "about a day") and that persist even when an organism (like a human) doesn't know the time of day.[1] As Jeremy Campbell explains in *Winston Churchill's Afternoon Nap*, a terrifically readable book on the human experience of time, "the body 'knows' what time of day or night it is, and so prepares itself for waking or sleeping, feeding and fasting. The changes going on inside the body keep a step ahead of the changes going on outside. This is a strategy for survival in evolution, as the use of a watch is a strategy for survival in business."[2]

Over the past few decades, chronobiologists have discovered innumerable patterns in the internal mechanisms that govern our appetite, temperature, blood pressure, cell division, hormone production, digestion, and every other process in our bodies. We have certain metabolic rhythms that govern how our bodies use calories, and we burn carbohydrates more effectively in the morning than we do at night. A given meal eaten every morning for a week may result in weight loss, while the identical meal eaten every evening for a week may cause weight gain. Studies show that the body uses dietary fuel differently at different times of day.[3] **Breakfast.** We have scrutinized the scientific literature about metabolic rhythms and have concluded that, although you process carbohydrates better in the morning, it's best not to break a night's fast with a food overload. Too big a breakfast will make anyone feel sluggish, and he or she won't be able to take advantage of the fact that peak intellectual capacity occurs during the morning hours. However, no breakfast at all may be even more disastrous for your body. As renowned cardiologist Michael DeBakey affirms, failure to break the night's fast will make your blood sugar levels crash, causing weakness, lethargy, concentration difficulties, headaches, or even nausea spells.[4] Plus you'll wind up overeating later in the day. For all of the above reasons, the *Double Your Energy With Half The Effort* diet includes plenty of recipes that make nutritious, quick-to-fix, light breakfasts and that tell the taste buds (and the rest of the body) to rise and shine. **Lunch.** The body handles food well at midday, and it needs slowly released energy to maintain performance over the afternoon. Of course, there's always the danger of sleepiness after a full lunch, but most people experience some sleepiness in the early afternoon regardless of what they've eaten. According to some scientists, this tendency is probably built into our systems; our ancestors slept during the middle of the day to avoid the hot sun. Our neighbors in Mexico and in Mediterranean and South American countries probably have the right idea: they pay attention to their circadian rhythms and enjoy rejuvenating *siestas* (naps) after their large midday meals. And take a look at little children; they often nap quite comfortably after their noon munch. Unfortunately, the American work day does not permit such pleasures as afternoon naps; however, a brief walk after lunch will do wonders to keep the brain in good working order. Plus you can use time after lunch to accomplish physical or routine tasks that don't require peak brain power. Research shows that mental capacity does increase again a few hours after a high-carbohydrate lunch.[5] If you eat most of your food fuel at lunch, you've got plenty of time to burn it off before bedtime. **Dinner.** Eating a light dinner late in the day eases your body into nighttime—and fixing a simple repast is much easier to face at the end of the day than preparing the conventional three- or five-course meal! Calories consumed at the close of the day simply don't burn that well. Your body doesn't need much energy to sleep, and your entire metabolism begins to slow down in the late afternoon. Meals that taste good, feel filling, yet don't contain a lot of calories make ideal suppers. For example, our *Sunsational Cinnamon Peaches, Tomatoes Montecito, Daniel's Meal-in-a-Muffin, Skinny Spuds, Millet San Marcos,* or any of our salads take just a few minutes to prepare, but they supply the crunch and flavor most of us crave after a hard day at the office or running around after kids. Plus these dishes give you energy to prepare food for tomorrow's hearty lunch as you straighten up the kitchen. **Snacks.** These need to be light, too. Sometimes our bodies and appetites tell us that an extra nosh is in order, so it's perfectly okay to snack on "uppers": fruits, vegetables, grain products, or any food that qualifies as nutritious and low in fat, sugar, and sodium. Carry snacks in your purse or briefcase so that you won't succumb to the temptations of vending machines or fast-food outlets. A packed snack can also come to the rescue of your energy levels when circumstances prevent you from eating a meal on time. No doubt you're aware that your brain's consciousness that it's mealtime triggers physiological responses that must be answered with food. (Think how often you've tried to muffle a growling stomach during an important appointment!) Thus healthy snacks play an important role in helping us to maintain high energy levels. So listen to your **internal cues**—physiological sensations of hunger, feelings of fatigue at odd times of day, dizziness, and so forth—and eat when you're truly hungry. Those internal cues, signals of your circadian rhythms, usually synchronize quite naturally with your brain's knowledge that it's time for breakfast, lunch, or dinner. And don't skip meals, or you'll throw the whole system off! Eating reasonable amounts of food at regular intervals will keep your whole body working smoothly and energetically. Become conscious of and begin to ignore **external cues** that tell you to eat at inappropriate times. When you do eat a meal or a snack, chew your food slowly and thoroughly, eat only in your kitchen or dining room, and focus completely on your food so that you can enjoy the texture, color, taste, and aroma of the food. Some people also benefit by arranging their meals attractively on small plates and using small utensils that prompt them to take more bites per serving. Eating while driving, sunning, working, reading or watching television will only sabotage your natural rhythms and condition your body to believe it needs food while you're engaged in those activities. And television advertisements provide far too many provocations to eat. As you're well aware, the media—and American society in general—encourages us to reward ourselves with food or alcohol for jobs well done. We celebrate almost every event by feasting. Of course, mild food splurges on holidays are understandable and may even be psychologically necessary, but food motivates too many of us on a daily basis, and some of us live to eat instead of the other way around.

Gaining control of your weight involves **modifying your behavior** so that you see food as the body fuel that it is rather than as a reward or security blanket. If you need to lose some pounds and fat, begin to substitute other appealing rewards for the food bonuses of which you're so fond. Try one of the following when you feel like patting yourself on the back, or even when you need a little cheering up:

- Take a leisurely drive or bike ride
- Call a friend or relative who lives far away
- Visit a museum, zoo, or amusement park

- Spend a night on the town—take in a concert, play, or movie
- Go dancing
- Rent a limousine and go for a luxury ride
- Get a new haircut or a manicure
- Get a massage or a facial
- Listen to a new recording or read a new book
- Spend a quiet evening propped up in bed and reading the stacks   of magazines you've been meaning to peruse
- Take an adult education course or sign up for music, art, or sports lessons
- Investigate and begin a new hobby
- Go shopping for clothes, shoes, or jewelry (if you can afford   them!)
- Visit the ocean or the nearest lake or river and spend an afternoon relaxing in the sunshine
- Plan and begin a new craft project
- Purchase some new exercise equipment or outfits
- Find yourself a pet and learn about its care and feeding
- Visit an elderly person who would love to see you
- Make a gift basket of toiletries or kitchen gadgets to give to a friend
- Plan a vacation
- Redecorate a room in your home
- Clean house—what seems like a chore may actually rejuvenate you

And while you're at it, begin a **food diary** in which you record absolutely everything you eat for at least a week. Include in your diary notations about what exactly prompted you to eat. An argument with a loved one or a boss? A spell of loneliness? Exhaustion after a long day? A salary raise? A birthday celebration? Just the process of writing down what goes into your mouth will make you think twice about food choices and amounts. Such a diary will also open your eyes as to your eating patterns and maybe even help you to perceive some of your body's circadian rhythms. Even though *Double Your Energy With Half The Effort* frees you to eat a whole range of fruits, vegetables, grains, and legumes almost indiscriminately, you'll be better equipped to withstand onslaughts of advertisements for packaged foods as well as the aromas of candy shops if you can motivate yourself to eat only what you've planned and only when you're truly hungry. One of the tricks to maintaining this kind of control of your diet is **visualization,** a simple technique by which you imagine a lean new you. Visualization involves daydreaming about the body you'd like to have. That's not too hard, is it? Fantasizing about yourself as a fashion model or a prize-winning athlete will help you set a positive goal for yourself and keep you from tossing your eating plan out the window. Place pictures of models or athletes or clothing you'd like to have on your refrigerator door to remind you of your resolve. Then visualize how good you'll feel about yourself tomorrow if you don't give in to temptation today. (But if you do succumb to a forbidden goodie, don't think you've blown your whole eating plan and start eating everything in sight! Simply visualize yourself back on track, eating piles of nutritious foods instead.)

One of the keys to sticking with the Light-Moderate-Light eating program and maintaining that positive image of yourself is **a kitchen well stocked with wholesome foods.** If you maintain a good inventory of good ingredients, you can cook almost anything you please at a moment's notice, and you won't have to run to the store every day, only to be tempted by packaged high-fat foods. Keep such unwholesome foods out of the pantry and refrigerator as well. If double-fudge brownies lurk in the cupboard, we'll bet they won't remain there but a day or two.

Below is a basic—but not exhaustive—list of ingredients vital to the *Double Your Energy* diet and to your kitchen. For greatest success with your new Light-Moderate-Light eating plan, keep a running list of those you need to replace. Prevent bare cupboards! (You'll find descriptions of less-familiar foods in the glossary at the back of this book.)

Flours and cereals: unbleached white flour, whole-wheat flour, yellow cornmeal, whole-grain pastry flour, wheat germ, oat bran, unprocessed wheat bran flakes, soy flour, bran cereal, oat cereal, millet, flax seeds.

Whole grains and related foods: barley, bulgur (cracked wheat), millet, rolled oats, brown rice, white rice, wild rice, pasta in all shapes and sizes (preferably the whole-grain variety).

Legumes, **dried and/or canned**: black beans, chickpeas (garbanzos), kidney beans, lentils, pinto beans, soybeans, split peas, white beans (navy or Great Northern), dry-roasted and unsalted peanuts.

Leavenings: baking powder, baking soda, cornstarch, active dry yeast.

Dried herbs and spices: allspice, basil, bay leaves, cayenne pepper, celery seed, chili powder, cinnamon, whole and ground cloves, coriander, cumin, curry powder, dillweed, garlic powder, ground ginger, kelp, marjoram, mint leaves, mustard powder, ground nutmeg, onion powder, oregano leaves, paprika, parsley flakes, black pepper, white pepper, poppy seeds, rosemary, savory leaves, shelled sesame seeds, tarragon, thyme leaves, commercial herb blends.

Liquid seasonings: almond extract, reduced-sodium soy sauce, Tabasco, tamari, tomato paste (no added salt), tomato sauce (no added salt), vanilla extract, vinegars, Worcestershire sauce.

Sweeteners: apple-juice concentrate, applesauce, honey, molasses (preferably blackstrap), raisins, maple syrup, rice syrup, dates, pineapple juice.

Oils: Cold-pressed safflower, sunflower, sesame, olive, peanut, corn.

Other necessary fats: butter (preferably the raw certified variety) or soft margarine (as unhydrogenated as possible), peanut butter, other nut butters. (Read the labels on containers of nut butter; avoid those butters that contain extra sodium or other additives.)

Dairy products: eggs; nonfat or low-fat milk, yogurt, and cottage cheese; hard cheeses.

Fresh vegetables: bean sprouts, broccoli and/or cauliflower, cabbage, carrots, celery, garlic, lettuce or spinach, mushrooms, onions (yellow or white), potatoes, tomatoes, plus whatever is in season.

Fresh fruits: apples, bananas, lemons, oranges, plus whatever is in season.

Condiments: ketchup (low-sodium), mustard, mayonnaise.

Other kitchen staples: powdered nonfat milk, nuts (walnuts, almonds), popping corn (the perfect snack food), soy milk, tofu.

Dining out. Stocking the shelves and dining at home are easy, you say. The recipes in *Double Your Energy With Half The Effort* are a cinch. You even plan your menus days ahead, and you can easily master the technique of preparing the next day's lunch the night before. So how do you handle meals away from home?

Because friends and menus may weaken your resolve to follow the Light-Moderate-Light meal plan, you'll especially need your powers of visualization when you dine out. Here are a few tips for coping with restaurant food:

• Eat an apple or a light snack before dining out so you won't feel ravenous and then eat impulsively.

• Order mineral water or fruit juice when your companions order alcohol. (See Chapter Two for our discussion of the dangers of alcohol.)

• Choose appetizers, soups, or salads that contain fresh fruits and vegetables, and request oil-and-vinegar, buttermilk, or yogurt dressings. Or simply use lemon juice to flavor your salad.

• Stick to the greens and fresh fruits offered at salad bars; avoid already-mixed salads like slaws, pasta salads, and bean salads that contain excessive amounts of oil and salt.

• Feel free to eat plenty of bread—but go easy on the butter.

• Order a la carte to avoid stomach overload.

• If you'd like an entré, choose a light pasta dish or

vegetables stir-fried in sesame or peanut oil. Avoid tempura or other deep-fried foods. If you feel the need to splurge, a little quiche or frittata should satisfy.

• Ask the waiter to hold the sauce; many restaurant-prepared sauces contain tons of cream and butter.

• Order fruit for dessert. Or go home to your own homemade desserts that contain less sugar and fat and higher quality carbohydrates than the restaurant variety. (For a wide array of healthy snack and dessert foods you can make yourself, take a look at our book *How to Survive Snack Attacks . . . Naturally.*)

• If portions are too big, take home a "doggie bag" of choice morsels.

Because restaurants all over the country are beginning to pay attention to the needs of health-conscious diners, many now offer "heart-healthy" dishes. And chefs at reputable eating establishments are certainly accustomed to requests from diners with special dietary needs. You're paying good money for the meal, so don't be afraid to ask for what you want! The longer you are able to follow the basic guidelines of the *Double Your Energy* diet, the easier it will be for you to turn down high-fat foods. Your retrained taste buds and your educated mind won't crave the foods that swell your body dimensions. And exercise (our next topic) will help you feel good about the way you look.

Chapter Four

Exercise: The Ultimate Energy Booster

When we tell you that exercise is absolutely essential to your success with the energy-raising *Double Your Energy With Half The Effort* diet, you wince. You already know that exercise is supposed to be good for you, but every time you start a new exercise program, your appetite seems to skyrocket. You assume that exercise is simply inviting bigger food bills and bigger bulges, and you tell yourself that physical activity will only make you feel more fatigued than usual. So you quit running or swimming or walking—or whatever sport you tried this time around.

Convincing your sedentary self that you've made the right decision seems especially easy after you hear proponents of crash diets proclaim that exercise in itself won't burn enough calories to make a dent in your excess fat. (And taking off one pound of flesh does require a lot of effort—about sixteen hours of bicycling or fast walking!) Advocates of quickie diets assert that the only way to lose weight is to eat fewer calories.

Trouble is, crash dieters, who may indeed lose weight quickly, tend to feel exhausted because they are depriving their bodies of food fuel. Furthermore, they simply pile the pounds back on when they return to their normal eating habits. Too often, perennial dieters pack on even more fat than they carried before their last diets. Fat propagates fat, and dieters who are temporarily successful but who normally carry too much fat will still tend to turn most of the food they eat into fat because they haven't developed any lean muscle tissue, the substance that works to remove body fat. As Jane Brody points out in her *Nutrition Book*, four out of five dieters who lose weight will eventually regain it. [1]

Low-calorie diets make our bodies fight to maintain what medical researchers now call the **set point**, the weight at which the human body stabilizes when its owner is not actively trying to gain or lose weight. When faced with calorie deficits, the area in our brains that regulates how much body fat we carry begins to panic, so it increases our appetites and clamps down our metabolisms so that we don't burn food calories or fat as well as we did before. Moreover, radical weight reduction diets can change body chemistries for the worse: although they will trigger weight loss, crash diets may actually raise set points and lower **basal metabolic rates**, the speed at which our bodies burn calories while we're at rest.

Yes, adhering to a lose-it-quick eating program lets you peel off pounds rapidly—but only at the diet's outset. The first weight to come off consists of water and muscle, body components much more easily shed than pounds of fat, each of which stores twice the number of calories as a pound of glycogen (carbohydrate storage) or protein. After the first five or ten pounds drop away, weight loss slows down, and your body struggles to conserve stored energy. You've got to have a lot of willpower to stick with a low-calorie diet for weeks on end. If you want to keep superfluous weight off, you may have to stay with the diet for years on end, too. But if you're like most dieters, you'll get pretty tired of limited food choices and calorie counting, and your body weight will bounce up and down as you diet, regain, diet, regain, *ad infinitum.*

But here's the flip side of the story: researchers have found in repeated studies that exercise improves body chemistry. Indeed, *exercise will lower your body's set point and raise your basal metabolic rate.* Even if you eat the same amount as you did before you began to exercise, you'll lose weight. No joke! Dr. Dennis Remington, an obesity expert at Brigham Young University, theorizes that the body somehow senses that an active person needs to be thin and lowers the body's set point.[2]

Now that you understand how physical exertion can transform your metabolism, give exercise an honest try. You'll notice that your appetite may decrease for a couple of hours after you exert yourself, and then increase an hour or two later. However, your body's lowered set point will give you a feeling of greater control over your appetite, and you'll burn off food calories more quickly than you did before. There's a bonus, too: Not only do you burn food calories and body fat during strenuous exercise, but *you continue to burn more calories than usual for hours after exercise because vigorous activity boosts your basal metabolic rate,* making it hard for your body to conserve energy in the form of fat. In fact, a team of scientists recently found that intense exercise stimulated calorie expenditure up to nine hours later, and lipid oxidation, or the burning of fat, for at least eighteen hours after the subjects had stopped exercising.[3]

And body fat is the issue here; losing anything other than body fat can be harmful. As Covert Bailey points out in his scientifically grounded, enormously popular book *Fit or Fat?* being overweight only signals that you are carrying too much fat, and those who think they maintain an ideal weight may be overfat, too.[4] The older you are, the more likely it is that your muscles have begun to turn to fat. The scales tell only a partial truth; the tape measure tells you a bit more. For example, two people who are the same age, weight, and height may look incredibly different in terms of fitness. One may be trim and muscular, and the other may exhibit rolls around the middle or pouches on the thighs. Part of the reason for this discrepancy in appearance is that the lean muscle on the first person weighs more than fat that pads the second. In addition, all bodies carry muscle in a neater fashion than they do fat.

Interestingly, researchers have proven that most heavy people don't eat more than thin people do; people who carry too much fat simply move less and have lower basal metabolic rates. Instead of using food fuel in vigorous movement, their bodies, which possess relatively little lean muscle, convert food fuel to fat. The only way that overly fat people can succeed at weight loss programs and then sustain a nearly ideal weight is to lower their set points and raise their metabolic rates permanently by involving themselves in a regular exercise program. How do you know if you're too fat? Don't rely on the scales. Take a look in the mirror; check to see if you've got padding where you don't want it. How do your clothes fit? Can you "pinch an inch" on the back of your upper arm? If you can, and you're a man, you're definitely packing too much fat. If you're a woman, you've probably got more than enough fat, too. For an even better assessment of your body composition, take advantage of the underwater immersion tests offered by fitness clubs or physicians. Such tests measure just exactly how much fat your body is hiding—or displaying. When you try an immersion test, remember that a healthy, lean man is 10-15 percent fat by weight, while a healthy, lean woman is about 15-20 percent fat. As we said in Chapter Two, every body needs fat to cushion organs, to metabolize certain vitamins, and to store energy for emergency purposes.

Drastically reducing your calorie intake will cause your

body to burn unnecessary fat eventually, but such deprivation saps energy and works against muscle gain. In contrast, exercising vigorously and regularly will pump up adrenaline levels and help you lose fat gradually and effectively. As we explained above, strenuous exercise creates the lean muscle that metabolizes fat all over your body. In case you didn't know it, there's no such thing as so-called spot reducing. You can tone up the muscles in a specific area, but the only way to lose fat in a certain spot is to exercise energetically.

Not all types of exercise qualify as fat reducers, however. The only kinds of exercise that will burn body fat are those that are **aerobic**, those that encourage the heart and lungs to use oxygen ("aero" is the Greek word for "air") steadily over a period of time. Aerobic exercise involves continuous movement of large muscle groups that send signals to the heart and lungs to circulate lots of oxygen. To get rid of excess body fat, you must perform aerobic exercise for at least 35 minutes at least four times a week. (That same exercise performed just three times a week will only maintain your fitness level.) For at least 20 of those minutes, your heart must be beating at its ideal training rate, which is between 70 and 85 percent of its age-determined maximum rate.

Sound too complicated? Actually, it's pretty simple to tell when you're exercising aerobically. Here's a formula to help you figure out your **maximum heart rate (MHR)**, the fastest your heart should ever beat:

$$\frac{220}{-\text{Age}}$$
maximum heart rate (MHR) per minute

Do *not* exercise at this rate. Instead, exercise so that your heart reaches its **training heart rate (THR)**, the ideal rate for burning body fat. To find both your minimum and maximum THR, take the MHR you calculated above and multiply it by both 70 percent and 85 percent:

$$\frac{\text{MHR}}{\times .70}$$
minimum training heart rate (THR) per minute

MHR

x .85

maximum training heart rate (THR) per minute

If your heart rate falls below your low-end figure, your muscles are not burning fat. If your heart rate exceeds a THR of 85 percent, you are exercising too hard and putting too great a strain on your heart. Paradoxically, exercising too intensely may cause muscle loss. To determine your heart rate at any time, put a couple of fingers in the groove next to your Adam's apple, or place your middle finger on your wrist at your pulse point. Count the beats for six seconds, and multiply by ten. (If you do this while you're exercising, keep your legs moving to keep your heart rate elevated.)

You can also tell whether you're exercising too hard by seeing if you can talk while you're in the middle of your chosen sport. If you've worked up a reasonable sweat and are breathing hard, but you can still talk to a companion, you're probably safely within your heart's training zone.

Practice figuring your heart rate as you do laundry, walk down the block to the bus, make the bed, mow the lawn, or whatever. You'll soon discover that all the hustle-bustle you thought was good exercise is not burning fat calories at all. The tasks you're performing are **anaerobic** ("without air") activities that may indeed strengthen and tone muscles, but that won't strengthen your cardiovascular system or increase your endurance. These exercises involve only short spurts of energy that don't sufficiently tax the lungs and heart. Included in the anaerobic group are such popular sports as weight lifting, tennis, football, baseball, skiing, golf, bowling, and sprinting.

Activities that can be aerobic, provided you perform them so that you achieve your THR for at least 20 minutes at least four times a week, include the following: **brisk walking, hiking, jogging, running, aerobic dancing, rowing, jumping rope, cross-country skiing, swimming, cycling, skating, soccer, basketball, racquetball, and handball.** Remember: movement in these types of exercise must be continuous. If you can maintain your training heart rate (THR) for 30 to 60 minutes, all the better. Normally, you need to exercise for at least 10 minutes before your muscles start working aerobically rather than anaerobically.

Aerobic exercise in which your body (not a machine) bears its own weight has added benefits especially for women; such sports help prevent osteoporosis by building muscles and increasing bone density. And when women couple weight-bearing exercise with menus from the *Double Your Energy* diet they significantly reduce their chances of developing osteoporosis because lacto-ovovegetarian diets also prevent bone mineral loss.[5]

We all make time to eat, so changing our diets doesn't seem to tax our schedules the way altering our fitness levels does. How can you find any time at all to exercise? You begin an exercise program slowly, and you gradually increase the frequency and duration of your workout times. You choose activities that appeal to you and that suit your age and pocketbook, and you vary your exercise menu so that you don't get bored. (If you are over 35 or have any medical problems, be sure to consult with a physician before embarking on a new exercise regime.) Once again, you need to listen to your circadian rhythms (discussed in Chapter Three) to find the time of day that will work best for you. Consider early morning or early evening workouts. If you're really aiming to lose fat rather than just to maintain your current fitness level, exercise before breakfast or at least two hours after your last meal; that way, your muscles will burn fat rather than the food you just ate. Or take a deserved exercise break right after lunch when you're feeling drowsy, and get your adrenaline pumping to rev up your system and activate your mind.

No matter which exercise you choose or what time of day you intend to do it, just be faithful to your plan. Remember to exercise aerobically at least four times a week for at least 35 minutes at a time. Those 35 minutes will allow you to warm up for about 10 minutes, maintain your training heart rate for 20, and then cool down for another 5 or 10 minutes. In addition to those 35 minutes, take a few minutes to perform some relaxed, non-bouncing stretches both before and after your regular workout. Stretching promotes flexibility and allows your muscles to ease into and out of demanding activities and prevents injury.[6] You may also wish to supplement aerobic exercise with muscle-building anaerobic exercise. Please note that it is wonderful if you commit to exercising, and we have found that exercising first thing in the morning gives one more energy during the day!

If you have trouble motivating yourself to exercise, find yourself a "body buddy" and make a pact to exercise together consistently. Join a fitness club or a community or office team; an upbeat environment and enthusiastic teammates will excite you about your sport. Or try buying and purchasing some snazzy workout outfits and shoes, and enjoy wearing them whenever you exercise.

After a few weeks on an aerobic exercise program, most people find that *exercise becomes addictive,* and 'they feel fatigued or depressed when they can't exercise. This beneficial addiction probably occurs because strenuous physical activity stimulates the production of beta-endorphin, a natural tranquilizer and pain-reducer that mimics the effects of morphine, the strong pain-killing narcotic. Because *regular aerobic exercise gives you a natural "high"* and helps to keep you relaxed but energetic, you are less likely to suffer from depression, anxiety, anger, and other everyday negative emotions. Furthermore, regular aerobic exercise dramatically improves the circulatory and elimination systems; decreases "bad" blood cholesterol by increasing the "good," HDL-transported cholesterol, a process we explained in Chapter Two; helps battle diabetes by lowering blood sugar levels; fights arthritis by enhancing the condition of joints; and improves sleep and increases daytime efficiency because it decreases anxieties and tensions.

But that's not all. Medical researchers continue to discover the ways in which aerobic exercise benefits our bodies and our minds. Paired with complex-carbohydrate menus like those in the *Double Your Energy,*diet consistently performed aerobic exercise will no doubt elevate your physical energy *and* enhance your mental efficiency in ways that scientists have not even documented yet.

Chapter Five

Maintaining Double Energy

Becoming a healthier person by eating well and exercising consistently may seem an agonizing procedure to those of you with potentially harmful habits. However, a willingness to take small, calculated steps rather than big, impulsive leaps toward the goal of double energy can make the process easy and pleasant. In fact, you'll become quite proud of the personal transformation you effect, and your gradually increasing energy will amply reward your efforts.

Nonetheless, we'll admit that acquiring and maintaining a large measure of physical energy takes more than simply eating nutritious complex carbohydrates and exercising aerobically and regularly. *Sustaining an energetic, exciting lifestyle also requires a positive view of life and of yourself, a willingness to change and to accept responsibility for your own health, an appreciation of other people, and an awareness of environmental hazards and benefits.*

A positive view of life and of yourself. You've heard plenty of clichés about positive mental attitudes, and you may simply ignore advice on this subject because it seems trite. Yet you can't succeed at any diet or plan for better living if you're the type who looks at any goal skeptically or who focuses on your failures rather than on what you've accomplished and what you can still achieve. And if you can't muster a sense of humor—if you can't summon a good, body-healing belly laugh now and then—your stress levels will probably become dangerous to your physical health.

You need to develop confidence in *Double Your Energy With Half The Effort* and in yourself if you want to multiply your physical energy and prevent disease. Harboring too many suspicions about the diet or thoughts that you might not succeed will program you for failure.

For example, a negative outlook inevitably sabotaged the noble intentions of a good friend of ours, who attempted a vegetarian diet several years ago at our prompting. After several weeks of meatless dining, he decided to call it quits. Because he believed that he was not getting any protein, he felt weak and tired. He had convinced himself that a meat-free diet would decrease rather than increase his energy. Had he learned that complex carbohydrates—not protein—are the body's first choice for energy production, he probably would have felt stronger and more alert than ever before. If he had been aware of the large number of high-caliber athletes who eat strictly vegetarian diets, he might have recognized his misconceptions about the relationship between animal protein and energy. Our friend's negative perception of vegetarianism had overruled his true physical sensations.

Developing a positive mental attitude about whatever project you've undertaken involves appreciating yourself and your capabilities. Focusing on the qualities you lack rather on your gifts will only undermine your efforts. Forget about comparing yourself to another person or to some image of perfection. Accept who you are now, and find ways to grow and improve. Loving yourself will free your mind to focus on your life's tasks—including increasing and then maintaining your energy.

We'll bet you know at least a few people whose feelings of inadequacy inhibit them every hour of every day. Unhappy with some aspect of their appearance or personality, they convey that dissatisfaction to other people, thereby influencing others to see them in the same way they see themselves. Full of inner turmoil, people with negative self-images tend to experience more than the usual number of conflicts in their personal relationships. In addition, their poor self-concepts make them feel more weary than they might otherwise. Almost every task tires them.

In contrast, those who possess self-confidence, who work on but simultaneously de-emphasize their own faults and failures, attract friends and admiration. Because they can laugh at and accept themselves, they often feel energetic and practically unconquerable. Such individuals create their own possibilities, and they make the perfect (but certainly not the only) recruits for the *Double Your Energy* diet. **Willingness to change and to accept responsibility for health.** Those who cannot accept themselves are often the same people who fear change or who believe themselves the victims of circumstance. Such individuals make poor candidates for any kind of diet or exercise plan. Furthermore, they are the people who succumb to serious illness when it strikes.

Many medical doctors have observed just how crucial a patient's attitude and flexibility are in healing him or her. You're probably familiar with human interest stories about people who have overcome critical illnesses almost by sheer force of will. Norman Cousins and his battle with a near-terminal illness is a prime example. Determined not to surrender to his disease, Cousins watched hours of Marx Brothers films and *Candid Camera* reruns, and he laughed his way to wholeness. He documents his miraculous journey back to health in the enormously popular *Anatomy of an Illness*.[1]

Dr. Bernie Siegel, a physician who works with terminally ill cancer patients, has likewise witnessed how individuals' willingness to change and to take responsibility for their health may prolong life or even save it. In his inspirational best seller titled *Love, Medicine & Miracles*, Siegel explains that "many people don't make full use of their life force until a near-fatal illness goads them into a 'change of mind.'" Part of this change usually involves learning to love of oneself:

> The fundamental problem most people face is an inability to love themselves, having been unloved by others during some crucial part of their lives. This period is almost always childhood, when our relations with our parents establish our characteristic ways of reacting to stress. As adults we repeat these reactions and make ourselves vulnerable to illness, and our personalities often determine the specific nature of the illnesses. The ability to love oneself, combined with the ability to love life, fully accepting that it won't last forever, enables one to improve the quality of life.[2]

Long before illness strikes, those who feel unloved and unlovely experience excessive fatigue. Negative images of themselves and feelings of helplessness make such people vulnerable to outside stresses and cause them to feel weary. Even if those same people are eating well and exercising regularly, their sense of hopelessness can negate their attempts to become healthy.

On the other hand, those who love themselves somehow recognize that potential for change lies inside them and that to some extent they can shape their worlds. Acceptance of self leads to interest in the world and to the realization that change is stimulating and challenging rather than frightening and dangerous. The individual who takes care of his or her body and who can see crises as opportunities for growth is a person whose energy levels will rise to meet whatever challenges he or she faces.[3]

If you are one who struggles with feelings of helplessness, or if you feel too comfortable with the status quo, at least begin to recognize the mental obstacles you've created for yourself. Perceiving a problem is half the struggle. When you can see negative emotions in yourself, you can address them and then release them. It's perfectly human and okay to feel bad about yourself once in a while, but experiencing chronic feelings of inadequacy can paralyze you.

Once you realize that you need to gain control of your life, take small steps toward enhanced appearance and health, increased energy, and greater happiness. What kinds of steps do we mean? In the case of dietary and exercise goals, altering ingrained habits can be painlessly simple if you attempt one modification at a time. For example, try substituting brown rice for your usual white rice. When you need a snack, eat an apple or a whole-grain cookie instead of a candy bar. Walk for a half hour during your lunch break; breathe deeply and notice your surroundings. When you've accepted a challenge once, try making that same change every other day—or every day. What was once different will become comfortably routine, and you will begin to sense the choices you can make about much larger aspects of your life.

An appreciation of other people. Accepting yourself and feeling in control of your own life will open your mind to love other people, and that love will energize your whole being and make you less vulnerable to illness.

Numerous studies have indicated that people who live in harmony with others experience far fewer bouts with disease and have greater longevity than those who feel in conflict with the world. For example, the landmark research that focused on the town of Roseto, Pennsylvania, showed that a strong sense of community, of belonging, was linked to a heart attack rate that was one-fourth the national average. Although citizens demonstrated all the high-risk factors—smoking, lack of exercise, and consumption of animal fat—their stable, supportive personal relationships diluted the effects of these bad habits.[4]

Harmonious personal relationships bring us all kinds of

energy. Skeptical? Just consider how far you'll travel to see a loved one, or how late you'll stay up to make something special for a favorite relative.

Now recall how your body usually feels when you're angry or resentful about another person's actions. Again, those emotions are perfectly natural, but you can learn to release them by making the other person aware of the problem and/or by recognizing that the other person's actions were actually masked requests for your love and attention. Of course, we're simplifying tremendously here, and you need to consult a counselor if you're carrying around a load of anger and resentment. Nonetheless, we can tell you that forgiveness, even if it is unspoken, is a powerful tool for healing and for regaining your own energy.

An awareness of environmental hazards and benefits. hanging yourself and relating positively with others may seem surprisingly easy compared to dealing with physical hazards over which we sometimes have little control. But once we become aware of potential problems—contaminated food or water and polluted air, for example—we can make choices that will better our lives and elevate our energy.

Learn where the produce you buy originates and how it is cultivated. Find out about your water supply and how its managers treat it chemically. Read about the level of pollutants in the air you breathe. If any of your discoveries troubles you, consider buying your food from natural foods stores or directly from organic growers; find an alternate drinking water supply (see our discussion of water in Chapter Two); and/or consider leaving an area in which the air carries excessive levels of pollutants. Do what you can to take charge of your health and that of other family members.

Breathing properly is important no matter which environmental hazards you face. The more deeply you breathe, the greater the amount of oxygen you send to your brain and the more energy you feel. The Chinese call the vital energy within each of us *chi*, and they call the art of manipulating one's breath *chi kung* ("inner vigor"), a discipline that reflects their belief that air fuels inner energy. You can learn what the Chinese have long practiced by taking classes in yoga, meditation, martial arts, or stress management.[5] Learning to breathe abdominally can bring all sorts of benefits, including a clear mind and an ability to relax quickly.

If you live in an area of excessive smog, you may want to invest in a filter or a negative ion machine for your home. *Ions* are electronically charged atoms or clusters of atoms. A positive ion *(cation)* results when a neutral atom or atom cluster loses an electron, which is a negatively charged particle; a negative ion *(anion)* results when an atom or atom cluster gains an electron. Pollution reduces the number of oxygen and hydrogen atoms available in the air, and it causes an imbalance in the ratio of negative and positive ions. Dry winds, like the Santa Anas here in California, carry an excess number of positive ions. Their presence makes people experience headaches, earaches, irritability, drowsiness, dry skin, and so forth. On the other hand, the presence of water, composed of hydrogen and oxygen atoms, indicates the existence of large numbers of negative ions, which scientists attribute with energizing properties.

If all this sounds too esoteric, remember how you've gotten flashes of insight while you were showering or before a rainfall, or how a vacation near a lake or ocean has made you feel particularly rejuvenated. Scientists need to investigate further the connection between negative ions, flowing water, and human energy, but you can nonetheless take advantage of energy-raising running water and negative ion machines right now.

In addition to exposing yourself to better air and more negative ions, you may also want to increase your energy by using a dry brush to massage yourself. Brushing your body, using a long-handled brush with natural vegetable bristles, removes dead skin cells and increases blood circulation all over your body, thereby encouraging your lungs to up your oxygen intake and thus to elevate your energy levels. Try dry-brushing once and see how you like it. Use long strokes that begin at your feet and legs and move up to your neck, and be sure that your brush is completely dry.

As you see from our discussion in this chapter, many different factors affect your energy quota and your spirits. Eating the "upper" foods and avoiding the "downer" foods described in Chapter Two of *Double Your Energy* following a Light-Moderate-Light daily eating plan (Chapter Three), and exercising aerobically and consistently (Chapter Four) can certainly double your energy and improve your health and appearance. However, to enjoy the full benefits of these life-changing practices, you need to accompany them with mental openness and a decision to grow in all facets of your life and personality. Such a conscious choice can lead not only to a personal transformation but to a transformation of the world around you.

PART II

Energizing Recipes

Eye-opening Applesauce
Yield: 1 serving

For a zippy breakfast in a bowl, begin with applesauce made from tart, freshly picked apples. The fruit and nuts contribute plenty of fiber; the raisins supply iron; and the wheat germ and brewer's yeast add minerals, B vitamins and protein.

1 cup unsweetened applesauce (see recipe for
 Instant Applesauce on page 242)
6 walnuts, diced
1-1/2 tablespoons wheat germ
1 tablespoon raisins
1 tablespoon brewer's yeast

Stir together and enjoy!

Paradise Pilaf
Yield: 4 Servings

Dried fruit virtually bursts with energy—producing nutrients—and with calories, too! Because it contains so much sugar, we use candy-like dried fruit sparingly, and we like to combine it with grains and other appetite-satisfying foods. In this recipe, the dried figs add pizzazz to spiced rice.

2 cups apple juice
1-1/2 cups water
1/2 cup dried figs (or dates, papaya, or pineapple), cut up
1-1/2 cups long-grain brown rice or wild rice
1/2 cup chopped celery
1 teaspoon thyme
1/2 teaspoon cinnamon
1/2 teaspoon nutmeg

Combine juice, water, and figs in a sauce pan and bring to

a boil. Stir in remaining ingredients, cover tightly, and continue to cook for 50 minutes.

Golden Pumpkin Muffins
Yield: 12 muffins

For the perfect autumn brunch, pair these pumpkin muffins with fresh fruit. Pumpkin is a super source of potassium, which helps you think clearly, and vitamin A, which keeps your skin looking as great as you feel.

1 egg, slightly beaten
1/2 cup milk
1/4 cup honey
1/4 cup sunflower or safflower oil
2/3 cup cooked or canned pumpkin
1/2 teaspoon cinnamon
1/2 teaspoon nutmeg
1/2 teaspoon allspice
1-3/4 cups whole-wheat flour
1/4 cup cornmeal
1/2 cup chopped pecans (optional)
1 teaspoon baking powder

Preheat oven to 400° F.

Grease a 12-cup muffin pan, or place fluted liners in each of the pan's muffin cups. Set aside.

In a medium bowl, combine egg, milk, honey, butter or margarine, pumpkin, cinnamon, nutmeg, and allspice.

In a small bowl, combine wheat flour and corn meal; add to egg mixture along with the pecans, if used. Stir just to moisten the dry ingredients; do not overmix.

Spoon batter into prepared muffin cups.

Bake 20 to 25 minutes or until golden brown. Serve warm.

Banana Breakfast Custard
Yield: 2 servings

A phenomenal source of high-quality protein, tofu combines beautifully with bananas. Make this silky custard before you go to bed tonight so that you're ready to eat and run tomorrow morning.

1/2 pound tofu
1 ripe banana
3 tablespoons thawed, unsweetened apple-juice   concentrate
1 tablespoon oil (preferably sunflower seed oil)
1 teaspoon vanilla extract
1 tablespoon shredded unsweetened coconut (optional)

Blend all ingredients until smooth. Add coconut, if desired. Pour the mixture into custard cups and chill thoroughly.

Beachside Blueberry Smoothie
Yield: 2 servings

We love to drink this healthy shake at the peak of the berry season. However, you can enjoy this healthy concoction all year 'round: simply buy an ample supply of fresh, whole berries when they're plentiful and freeze the berries in zip-close bags.

1 ripe banana, sliced
1 cup fresh blueberries (or strawberries)
1/2 cup crushed ice
1 tablespoon brewer's yeast

Purée all the ingredients in a blender. Serve garnished with a few fresh blueberries or sliced strawberries.

Carob Fudge Balls
Yield: 50 (1/2-inch) balls

These confections make super breakfasts or snacks on-the-go. Pack them in a knapsack or handbag, and enjoy your meal on the road.

3 tablespoons honey (optional)
1 cup warm water
2 cups dry-roasted, unsalted sunflower seeds
1/2 cup pitted dates, diced
3/4 cup carob powder (roasted)
1 tablespoon vanilla extract
1 teaspoon cinnamon

Dissolve the honey in water.
Place the sunflower seeds in a blender or food processor and whirl until they become about 1-1/2 cups of powdery meal.
Combine sweetened water and sunflower-seed meal with the other ingredients, mix well, and roll the mixture into bite-size balls.

Note: Make these Carob Fudge Balls look especially attractive by rolling them in shredded unsweetened coconut.

Summerland Sunflower Cookies
Yield: 3-1/2 dozen cookies

We believe that breakfasts should be tempting and varied, so we have included this cookie recipe in our breakfast section. However, you can enjoy these energizing, high-protein, high-iron cookies any time. (We often reach for them when we feel one of our notorious late-night snack attacks coming on.)

1/3 cup honey
1/4 cup sunflower or safflower oil
2 eggs, beaten
3/4 cup dry-roasted, unsalted sunflower seeds, shelled
1/4 cup whole-wheat flour, sifted

5 tablespoons carob powder
1 teaspoon vanilla extract

Preheat oven to 350° F.
Blend honey, oil, and eggs.
Mix in flour, carob powder, sunflower seeds, and vanilla extract.
Drop by teaspoonfuls onto a lightly oiled cookie sheet.
Bake for 10 minutes, or until cookies appear lightly browned.

Note: Adding one ripe, mashed banana to the dough will give your cookies a tropical twist.

Sunsational Cinnamon Peaches
Yield: 1 or 2 servings

Nothing beats the taste of fresh, ripe peaches eaten out of hand. Nonetheless, fresh peaches also make a scrumptious hot breakfast that will satisfy an early-morning sweet tooth naturally.

2 large, ripe peaches, sliced
1/2 cup water
1 teaspoon ginger
1 tablespoon lemon juice
1 tablespoon raisins
1 tablespoon honey
1 teaspoon cinnamon
Dash of nutmeg

Preheat oven to 350° F.
Place peaches in a small baking dish.
Combine cinnamon, water, ginger, lemon juice, raisin, and honey; pour the mixture over the peaches.
Sprinkle with nutmeg and bake for 15 minutes.

Carpinteria Cranberry Bread
Yield: 2 loaves

Surprise overnight guests: adorn a breakfast table with seasonal flowers, freshly squeezed juices, fresh fruit, and slices of this colorful, fragrant bread. (Be sure to freeze several bags of cranberries when they're in season so that you can make these delectable loaves any time you please.) The whole-grain pastry flours help to give these loaves a fine, moist texture.

2 oranges
2 cups whole-wheat flour
2 cups whole-wheat pastry flour (or soy flour)
1 teaspoon baking powder
1 teaspoon baking soda
1-1/2 cups honey
1/2 cup chopped nuts
2 cups chopped or sliced cranberries
1/2 cup raisins
3 egg whites

Preheat oven to 325° F.

Grate the rind off the oranges and reserve rind. Cut each orange in half and squeeze out the juice. Add enough boiling water to juice to make 1-1/2 cups liquid.

Stir together the dry ingredients, and combine with the juice, rind, honey, oil, nuts, cranberries, and raisins.

Beat the egg whites just until they form stiff, moist peaks. Fold into batter.

Spread batter in two lightly oiled 9" x 5" loaf pans. Bake for one hour or until wooden pick in center comes out clean.

Crispy Rice Spice
Yield: 1 serving

When dousing our cold breakfast cereals, we often prefer juice to milk. Juices contain no fat, and they provide a change of pace, vitamins, and just the right touch of sweetness. The dates in this recipe pack lots of sugar for their small size, but they're also great sources of iron and other energy-raising nutrients.

1 cup crispy rice cereal with no salt
3/4 cup apple juice
dash cinnamon
3 dates, sliced
Combine all ingredients, and eat as a cold cereal.

Oat Float
Yield: 1 serving

Here's a deliciously simple way to take the humdrum out of breakfast fare.

1-1/4 cups oat ring cereal or 1 cup cooked oatmeal
1/2 cup apple juice or sparkling apple cider
2 tablespoons walnuts, diced
1 tablespoon raisins
1 tablespoon brewer's yeast (optional)

Place cereal in a bowl and add apple juice, walnuts, raisins, and brewer's yeast. Eat and enjoy!

Variation: Substitute bran cereal or puffed grain cereal for oats.

Los Padres Granola
Yield: 6 servings

This granola is our absolute favorite breakfast cereal and trail food. However, the tempting combination of high-fiber grains, seeds, and nuts does contain a fair number of calories and fat (the unsaturated variety), so we dole it out sparingly. You'll love it for those mornings when your body needs a little extra encouragement to get moving.

1/2 cup honey (or 1/2 cup maple syrup or rice syrup)
2/3 cup safflower oil
2 pounds rolled oats
2 cups diced almonds
2 cups shelled sunflower seeds
1 cup sesame seeds
1 cup wheat germ
1/2 cup chopped cashews
1/2 cup dried apricots (optional)

Preheat oven to 350° F.
Place honey and oil into a large pot and heat through.
Remove from heat, stir in dry ingredients, and mix well.
Spread mixture over cookie sheets and bake for 12 minutes, stirring occasionally.

Summer Solstice Muffins
Yield: 60 muffins

Each June, our city celebrates the beginning of summer with an unusual parade consisting of masked, costumed revelers. The evening before the zany spectacle, we mix up the batter for these chewy, moist muffins, and store the batter in the refrigerator. Then, on parade morning, we bake plenty of muffins to share with our favorite participants and spectators. If we have any muffins left over (a rarity), we freeze them in anticipation of our next weekend brunch.

2 cups boiling water
1 tablespoon baking soda
1 cup oil
3/4 cup honey
6 egg whites
4 cups Grape Nuts™ cereal or Los Padres Granola
2 cups bran flakes cereal
5 cups whole-wheat pastry flour
1 quart buttermilk
1/2 cup walnuts, diced
3/4 cup raisins
1/2 cup diced pineapple

Mix baking soda and boiling water. Set aside to cool.

Cream together oil and honey. Add egg whites and mix well.

Combine Grape Nuts™ cereal and flour. Add to creamed mixture along with buttermilk. Add water and baking soda mixture. Stir in walnuts and raisins. Mix well.

When you're ready for muffins, preheat oven to 375° F. Stir the pineapple into the batter, and spoon into lightly oiled or paper-lined muffin tins. Return extra batter to the refrigerator.

Bake muffins for 20-25 minutes or until toothpick inserted in center comes out clean. Serve immediately.

Surf's Up Soyuncream
Yield: 6 servings

This cool, creamy blend of protein-packed ingredients may seem almost like a dessert. Nonetheless, it makes a terrific—and unusual—breakfast, particularly on a warm morning. Because you make Soyuncream from soy milk, even those who have milk allergies can enjoy the tasty concoction. Plus the flax seeds provide exceptionally effective fiber for your digestive tract.

2 cups soy milk
1 cup raw almonds
1 cup pecans, toasted
1 cup shelled sunflower seeds
1/4 cup flax seeds
1/2 cup honey
1/4 cup safflower of sunflower oil
1 tablespoon vanilla
1 tablespoon shredded coconut

Whirl all ingredients in an electric blender until smooth. Pour into six small cups or into an ice-cube tray and chill thoroughly.

Sunup Pudding
Yield: 2 servings

Particularly appealing to kids, this wholesome yogurt "pudding" whips up in a jiffy, and it satisfies a body's morning requirements for calcium, vitamin C, and fiber.

1-1/2 cups plain nonfat or low-fat yogurt
1/2 cup wheat germ
6 tablespoons thawed unsweetened orange-juice concentrate
2 tablespoons thawed unsweetened apple-juice concentrate
4 tablespoons diced papaya
3 tablespoons crushed pineapple
1 tablespoon brewer's yeast (optional)

Purée or beat all ingredients except the pineapple.
Pour into custard cups and sprinkle with crushed pineapple.
Serve immediately.

Riviera Lift
Yield: 1 serving

A nice departure from run-of-the-mill breakfast cereal, this concoction will satisfy anyone's cravings for chewy, crunchy, or sweet foods. The recipe combines vitamin C (pineapple) with iron (raisins), protein (sunflower seeds, bran, brewer's yeast), potassium (banana) and vitamin A (applesauce). Plus the ample helping of brewer's yeast will aid your body in handling the day's stresses.

1 banana, sliced
1/2 cup unsweetened pineapple chunks
1/2 cup applesauce
2 tablespoons dry-roasted, unsalted sunflower seeds
2 tablespoons brewer's yeast
1 tablespoon raisins
1 tablespoon bran

Combine all the ingredients and serve.

Beach Banana-Oat Bread
Yield: 1 loaf

Try this simple but scrumptious loaf on a lazy weekend morning when you've got plenty of time to enjoy its flavor and texture. There's a bonus hidden in each slice: the bread's valuable fiber will help to lower the cholesterol in your blood.

1 cup raisins
1 cup rolled oats
1 1/2 cup whole-wheat pastry flour
1 cup bran
1 teaspoon cinnamon
1/4 teaspoon nutmeg
3 ripe bananas, mashed
1 cup milk
1/2 cup honey
1/2 cup walnuts
2 eggs, beaten

Preheat oven to 350° F.

Mix milk, honey, bananas, and eggs together.
With a wooden spoon, stir together dry ingredients, and then add them slowly to the liquid ingredients. Stir in remaining ingredients.
Spoon the mixture into a lightly oiled or buttered loaf pan and bake for one hour or until a wooden toothpick inserted in center comes out clean.
Cool the loaf in the pan for 10 minutes, and then turn it out onto a cooling rack.
Serve warm or at room temperature.

Coyote Corn Bread
Yield: 24 squares

Not only does this moist corn bread make a great breakfast item, but it tastes great with our Gaucho Baked Beans or alongside (or even crumbled into) any kind of salad or soup. Sunny yellow cornmeal contains far more vitamin A than does the white variety.

5 cups yellow cornmeal
2 cups whole wheat flour, sifted, or whole-wheat pastry flour
1/4 cup dry millet (optional)
1 tablespoon baking powder
4-5 cups buttermilk (or mix 4 cups of water with 2 cups of
plain nonfat yogurt)
3/4 cup honey
3/4 cup safflower oil
1 ear corn, kernels cut off
2 cups carrots, diced
1/4 cup diced chilies

Preheat oven to 325° F.
In a large bowl, stir together cornmeal, flour, millet, and baking powder. Add remaining ingredients, stirring just until moistened.
Spoon mixture into lightly greased 9" x 13" pan.
Bake for about 45 minutes to one hour.

Santa Ynez Apple Muffins
Yield: 24 muffins

Santa Ynez Valley orchards, which lie just a few miles north of Santa Barbara, grow the crispy apples we like to include in these moist, spicy, high-fiber muffins, which remind us of autumn and the holidays.

1 cup oil
4 eggs, beaten
2-1/2 cups whole-wheat pastry flour
1/2 cup bran
2 tablespoons cornmeal
2 teaspoons baking powder (optional)
2 teaspoons cinnamon
3/4 teaspoons nutmeg
1/2 teaspoon allspice
1-1/2 teaspoons vanilla
3/4 cup chopped walnuts
3/4 cup raisins
2 large apples, peeled, cored, and grated

Preheat oven to 400° F.

In a large bowl, combine honey, oil, and eggs.

Stir together the dry ingredients, and then add them, along with the vanilla, walnuts, raisins, and apples, to the honey mixture. Stir only until all the ingredients are moistened.

Spoon into oiled or paper-lined muffin pans, filling each cup about 2/3 full.

Bake for 35-45 minutes.

Santa Maria Strawberry Bread
Yield: 4 servings

Rich in vitamin C and potassium, strawberries taste wonderful in just about everything, including bread! Fresh strawberries are available in markets almost year-round now, so you can indulge in this unusual but addictive bread whenever you want.

1/2 cup unsweetened apple juice concentrate
1 egg
1/3 cup milk
1-1/4 cup whole-wheat flour
1/2 cup wheat germ
1 cup strawberries, sliced
1/2 cup filberts or pecans

Preheat oven to 325° F.

Combine ingredients in the order given and spread in a 9" x 5" loaf pan.

Bake for approximately one hour, or until toothpick inserted in center comes out clean.

Ortega-Ridge Orange Muffins
Yield: 24 muffins

Full of fiber and calcium, these goodies will boost your energy and your spirits. Try adding orange rind to the batter to give the muffins an extra bit of zingy orange flavor.

3 eggs, beaten
1 egg white, beaten until stiff
3 cups plain nonfat or low-fat yogurt
1 cup molasses
3/4 cup honey
1/2 cup safflower oil
   juice from two oranges (approximately half a cup total)
4 cups whole-wheat flour
1 tablespoon baking soda (optional)
1 tablespoon cinnamon
1 teaspoon nutmeg
1 cup raisins
3/4 cup toasted sunflower seeds
1 tablespoon orange rind (optional)
1 teaspoon vanilla

Preheat oven to 350° F.
Beat together all liquid ingredients.
In a separate bowl, stir together flour, bran, baking soda, and spices.
Slowly stir dry ingredients into liquid ingredients. Add raisins, sunflower seeds, orange rind, and vanilla extract.
Spoon into paper-lined or lightly oiled muffin pans, filling each cup about 2/3 full.
Bake 20-30 minutes, or until golden brown and tops spring back when touched lightly.

Wholesome Whole-Wheat Pancakes
Yield: 12 medium-sized pancakes

There's practically nothing more satisfying than eating pancakes for breakfast. The protein-building amino acids in the soy flour complement those in the wheat flour, so these pancakes pack plenty of protein.

3/4 cup whole-wheat flour (pastry flour)
1/4 cup soy flour
3/4 cup water
1 egg, beaten
2 tablespoons honey
1 tablespoon oil

1 teaspoon vanilla

Stir together all ingredients.

For each pancake, pour a large tablespoon of batter on a lightly greased and moderately hot frying pan or griddle. Cook each pancake until bubbles appear on the top and the bottom is golden. Flip, and cook until the other side is golden, too.

Serve with maple syrup, pecans, nonfat or low-fat yogurt, or fresh fruit.

Additional Breakfast Hints

1. Mix 1/4 cup water, 3 tablespoons rolled oats, dried fruit (raisins, currants, or chopped apricots), and/or seeds (pumpkin, sunflower, chia). Let the mixture stand overnight. In the morning, top with fresh fruit and enjoy!

2. Make a small but eye-appealing fruit salad to eat at breakfast.

3. Stir together applesauce and bran and/or brewer's yeast.

4. For a change of pace and a protein lift, pour soy milk instead of dairy milk over your cold cereal. The soy milk and whole grains create complete protein.

Anacapa Antipasto
Yield: 6 servings

What a terrific munch for lunch! This is the Santa Barbara version of traditional antipasto, that terrifically satisfying— but highly salted—Italian appetizer. (If you're watching your sodium intake, omit the olives from our second selection of vegetables.) We usually make lots of either antipasto version because it stays fresh in the refrigerator for up to three days.

Fresh, traditional vegetables (Group 1)

6 cups chopped cauliflower
4 cups chopped broccoli
2 cups diced carrots
1-1/2 cups diced zucchini
1 medium-sized, green bell pepper, seeded and chopped

Classic Italian vegetables (Group 2)

1 pint cherry tomatoes
1/2 pound fresh mushrooms, sliced thickly
1 medium-sized, red bell pepper, seeded and chopped
2 green onions, chopped
1/2 of a 13- ounce jar of medium-hot chili peppers, drained
1 can (6 ounces) pitted black olives, drained
1 can (6 ounces) artichoke hearts, drained and quartered

Dressing

1/2 cup tomato-based chili sauce
1/4 cup freshly squeezed lemon juice
1/4 cup wine vinegar
1 tablespoon olive oil
2-3 cloves garlic, minced
1 teaspoon oregano leaves
1 teaspoon basil
1/2 teaspoon dry mustard
pinch dried parsley

Prepare the vegetables in Group 1 or Group 2. If you choose the vegetables in Group 1, parboil each vegetable separately so that each maintains a little crispness. Drain.

In a large bowl, combine the vegetables in either group.

In a saucepan, combine all the dressing ingredients and bring them to a boil.

Immediately pour the hot dressing over the vegetables.

Toss vegetables gently, cool to room temperature, and then pour off excess dressing (and save if you wish).

Chill vegetable mixture thoroughly.

Speedy Sprice Sandwich
Yield: 3 servings

Naturally, we love sandwiches made on whole-grain breads. However, we occasionally feel like something crunchier and less caloric than bread, so we make a meal of crispy rice cakes spread with taste-tempting toppings. The texture of these applesauce "sandwiches" is particularly appealing.

6 rice cakes
3/4 cup applesauce
1 teaspoon cinnamon
1/2 teaspoon nutmeg
1 apple, peeled and grated
1/2 cup raisins
1/2 cup walnuts, diced
6 thin slices of Monterey jack cheese (optional)

Mix applesauce with cinnamon and nutmeg.

Spread about one tablespoon of applesauce on each rice cake, and top with shredded apple, raisins, and walnuts.

If you wish, place a cheese slice on top of the other ingredients and place cakes under a broiler only until the cheese melts.

Shoreline Shell Salad
Yield: 3 servings

The dressings on commercially made pasta salads often contain far too much fat, so we like to mix up our own low-fat, high-carbohydrate salads in the evening and chill them until lunch the next day. (Pasta salads require little preparation time, and they keep well in the refrigerator for several days.) If asparagus are not in season when you want to concoct this colorful salad, substitute broccoli or another fresh green vegetable cut into bite-sized pieces.

8 ounces small pasta shells
1/2 pound fresh asparagus
1 green onion, sliced thinly
1 cup cherry tomatoes, halved
1 carrot, diced
2 tablespoons olive oil
1/4 cup cider vinegar
1 teaspoon dried basil leaves
1 teaspoon dried parsley flakes
lettuce leaves
1/2 cup toasted almonds or raw walnuts

Boil pasta according to package directions or until al dente. Drain and rinse with cold water. Set aside in a large bowl.

Clean and trim asparagus spears, and then cut into one-inch pieces. Steam until the pieces are tender.

Add asparagus to pasta, along with onion, tomatoes, carrot, oil, vinegar, herbs, and nutmeg. Toss gently to distribute ingredients.

Chill salad for at least two hours so that flavors can blend.

Arrange lettuce leaves attractively on plates, top with pasta salad, and garnish with nuts.

Mushrooms Arlington
Yield: 4 servings

This gourmet entrée takes a little preparation time, but for a special luncheon, the work is well worth it. Because avocados are higher in fat and calories than practically any other fruit or vegetable, we indulge in "alligator pears" only occasionally. However, the fat in avocados is unsaturated oil, and the fruit's luscious flesh also contains vitamins A and C, folic acid, potassium, and niacin.

1 bunch fresh spinach
2 tablespoons butter
16 large mushrooms (each about 2" in diameter)
1 garlic clove, crushed
1 hard-boiled egg, chopped
1 teaspoon prepared mustard
1 teaspoon dried thyme leaves
1 teaspoon ground pepper
2 tablespoons mayonnaise
1 tablespoon sour cream
1/4 cup grated Parmesan cheese (about 3/4 ounce)
2 ripe avocados, mashed

Wash fresh spinach thoroughly and chop. Set aside.

Remove mushroom stems and chop finely.

In a medium skillet, melt raw butter. Add chopped mushroom stems and garlic. Sauté until the stems are soft; remove from heat. Add chopped spinach, hard-boiled egg, mustard, thyme, pepper, mayonnaise, sour cream, cheese, and avocado.

Preheat oven to 350° F.

Stuff each mushroom cap with spinach and avocado mixture, and place mushrooms, stuffed sides up, in an 11" x 7" shallow baking pan. Pour 3/4 cup water into the bottom of the pan and around the mushrooms, taking care not to pour water on top of the mushrooms.

Bake 20 minutes or until mushrooms are hot. (Check pan once or twice to be sure the water has not boiled away.)

Remove mushrooms from pan and discard any remaining liquid. Serve immediately.

Surfside Stroganoff
Yield: 6 servings

Ladled over bulgur, whole-wheat pasta, or brown rice, this

stroganoff will satisfy the voracious appetites of wind surfers, snorkelers, swimmers—and harried office workers, too. Plus a grain coupled with beans provides complete protein that may actually reduce the cholesterol levels in your blood.

1 teaspoon oil
2 cups chopped mushrooms
1 large onion, sliced
1 clove garlic, minced
1/4 cup whole-wheat flour
1 cup Nanya's Vegetable Stock, page 208, or water
4 teaspoons Worcestershire sauce
1/8 teaspoon marjoram leaves
1/8 teaspoon chili powder
1/8 teaspoon thyme leaves
2-1/2 cups cooked pinto beans or 2 cans (16 ounces each)
   pinto beans, drained (use low-sodium, if available)
1-1/2 cups plain low-fat yogurt
1 teaspoon freshly squeezed lemon juice
1/2 cup mayonnaise
6 cups cooked bulgur, rice, or noodles

Heat the oil in a large skillet, and add the mushroom, onion, and garlic. Sauté until tender.

Combine flour, vegetable stock, Worcestershire sauce, herbs, and spices; add to onion mixture in skillet and simmer until thickened. Add beans, and stir over low heat until beans are heated through.

Remove skillet from heat and stir in yogurt, lemon juice, and mayonnaise. Serve over bulgur, rice, or noodles.

East Beach Broccoli Quiche
Yield: 4-6 servings

Rich in vitamins A and C, low-calorie broccoli also offers active bodies a good dose of protein, iron, and calcium, and it probably helps prevent cancer. Broccoli tastes terrific all by itself, but it may taste even better when complementing potentially rich ingredients like cheese and eggs. Named for a local area where broccoli grows abundantly, this hearty midday meal also makes a great hors d'oeurve or supper entrée.

18" whole-wheat pie crust, purchased or made
  from our Whole-Wheat Pie Crust recipe (page 244)
1 medium onion, chopped
1 clove garlic, minced
6 large mushrooms, sliced
1 medium bunch broccoli, cut into flowerets
  and 1/4" slices of stem (approximately 2 cups)
4 eggs, beaten
1 cup milk
2 tablespoons brewer's yeast
1/2 teaspoon nutmeg
1/2 teaspoon dried basil leaves
dash cayenne pepper
1 cup grated Monterey jack cheese
1/2 cup grated Parmesan cheese

Preheat oven to 350°.

Place onions, mushrooms, broccoli and garlic on the bottom of the pie crust.

In a large bowl, beat the eggs. Stir in the milk, brewer's yeast, nutmeg, basil, and cayenne.

Pour the egg mixture over the vegetables, sprinkle the cheeses on top, and bake at 350° for 45 minutes or until a knife inserted in the center comes out clean.

County Bowl Cabbage Rolls
Yield: 4 servings (16 rolls)

Cabbage needn't bore you! Sweet-tasting cooked cabbage makes a great foil to spicy ingredients and provides good dietary fiber. The tofu and brown rice in this recipe pack all the protein you'll need for a busy afternoon.

2 small heads cabbage

Sauce

1 large onion, chopped
3 cans (8 oz. each) unsalted tomato sauce
1/2 teaspoon ground ginger
1/4 cup honey

1/4 cup vinegar
1/4 teaspoon thyme leaves
pepper to taste

Filling

1 large onion, chopped
1 stalk celery, diced
8 ounces tofu, cut into small cubes
1/2 cup chopped fresh parsley
1/2 cup unsalted tomato paste
2 cups cooked brown rice
1/4 teaspoon garlic powder

Remove the core from each cabbage, and steam cabbage heads for 20 minutes. Cool, and then carefully separate the leaves.

Prepare sauce: Steam chopped onion until translucent, and then place onion in a saucepan. Add remaining ingredients and simmer gently for about 30 minutes.

Preheat oven to 350°.

Prepare filling: Steam the chopped onion until translucent, and place the onion in a saucepan. Add remaining ingredients and heat thoroughly. Place about one tablespoon of the filling on each cabbage leaf, roll up tightly, and secure with a wooden toothpick.

Assemble dish: Place a small amount of sauce in a shallow baking pan (9" x 13" will do) and add the cabbage rolls. Pour remaining sauce over the rolls. Cover pan and bake for 45 minutes to one hour, or until the cabbage is soft.

Garnish with additional parsley, if desired.

Gaucho Baked Beans
Yield: 8 cups

Dark, sweet, and flavorful, these baked beans remind us of a country picnic—and they furnish our bodies with lots of protein, B vitamins, and calcium. Eat some fresh tomatoes with this soul-satisfying dish, and the tomatoes' vitamin C will help your body to absorb all the valuable iron the beans contain.

1 pound cooked navy beans
2 onions, chopped
1/2 cup ketchup
1/3 cup dark molasses
2 tablespoons honey
1 teaspoon dry mustard
boiling water as needed

Preheat oven to 325°.
Combine ingredients in a two-quart casserole. Add enough boiling water to cover bean mixture. Cover the casserole and place it in the oven. Bake for five to six hours, adding more boiling water if needed.

Calle Real "Creamed" Vegetables
Yield: 4 servings

Here is a low-fat, low-calorie version of a traditional, rich vegetable dish. Our rendition whips up quickly and gives you a midday helping of fiber, calcium, and vitamins. Be sure to use a variety of vegetables to please the palate and the eye.

4 cups vegetables (e.g., broccoli, carrots, cauliflower,
  onions, potatoes, turnips), cut into bite-size pieces
1-1/2 tablespoons safflower margarine
1-1/2 tablespoons whole-wheat or unbleached flour
1/2 teaspoon nutmeg (optional)
1/4 teaspoon pepper (optional)
1 teaspoon no-sodium vegetable seasoning
1-1/2 cups nonfat milk

Steam vegetables until barely tender. Drain well.
While vegetables are cooking, melt margarine in a medium-sized saucepan over low heat.
Add flour, nutmeg, pepper, and salt. Stir constantly over low heat until mixture is smooth. Remove from heat. Add milk and heat to boiling, stirring constantly for about one minute, or until mixture thickens.
Add cooked, drained vegetables and continue simmering mixture until vegetables are heated through.

El Colegio Curried Cauliflower
Yield: 4 servings

If you've a hankering for a hot lunch that's gooey and chewy—and inexpensive—here's the perfect dish. cancer-preventing cauliflower provides potassium and vitamin C; the other ingredients in this recipe offer you complete protein plus quality carbohydrates to fuel your afternoon efforts.

1 head cauliflower
1 tablespoon oil
1 medium onion, chopped
4 cloves garlic, minced
1/4 cup whole-wheat flour
1-1/2 cups water
1/2 cup skim milk
1 teaspoon curry powder (or more, to taste)
1/2 teaspoon ground ginger
1/4 teaspoon celery seed
1/2 cup raisins
1 cup shredded Monterey jack cheese (try low-fat)
2-4 cups cooked spinach noodles or rice
1 cup plain yogurt as a condiment (optional)

Wash cauliflower and cut into flowerets (about 5 cups). Stem flowerets until barely tender.

Heat oil; add onions and garlic. Saut_ until tender. Add flour and stir until blended. Add water and milk; cook and stir with a wire whisk until mixture has thickened. Add seasonings and mix well. Add raisins, cheese, and drained cauliflower, and stir until cheese melts.

Serve cauliflower mixture over spinach noodles or rice, and accompany with plain nonfat or low-fat yogurt, if desired.

Egg-ceptional Eggplant Parmesan
Yield: 4 servings

This traditional Italian dish pairs calcium-rich cheeses with adaptable eggplant, a high-fiber vegetable that absorbs other foods' flavors beautifully.

1 large eggplant (or 2 small eggplants)
  shallow bowl of very warm water
2 eggs, beaten
1/2 cup plain nonfat or low-fat yogurt
1/2 cup water
1 cup bread crumbs
12 oz. tomato sauce
2 cloves garlic, minced
1 teaspoon dried basil
1 teaspoon dried parsley
1 teaspoon dried Italian herb blend (optional)
1/2 cup sliced mushrooms
1/8 cup sliced black olives
3/4 cup shredded part-skim mozzarella cheese
1/2 cup shredded Monterey jack or cheddar cheese
1/2 cup grated Parmesan cheese

Preheat oven to 350° F.

Completely or partially peel the eggplant and slice crosswise into 1/2" slices. Soak the slices in warm water for 20 minutes and then drain.

In a wide bowl or dish, combine eggs, yogurt, and water. Dip eggplant slices in this mixture, and sprinkle both sides of each slice with bread crumbs.

Place breaded slices in a large casserole.

Stir together tomato sauce, garlic, herbs, mushrooms, and olives. Spread evenly over eggplant slices.

Distribute shredded cheeses on top of slices, and sprinkle with Parmesan. If you wish, pour any leftover egg mixture on top or around the eggplant slices.

Bake for about 45 minutes or until slices seem tender when poked with a fork.

West-side Enchilada Casserole
Yield: 8 servings

These enchiladas are so easy to make, and you will get so many compliments.

**8 large no-lard flour tortillas
1 large jar of picante sauce (medium heat)
1 bunch of chopped green onions (scallions)
1 clove garlic minced
1 can of sliced black olives
1 large red bell pepper, diced
1 can sliced mushrooms
1 8-ounce box of low-fat cream cheese
2 cups of shredded Monterey Jack cheese
1/2 cup of shredded Monterey Jack cheese for sprinkling on top**

Preheat oven at 350°F.

Beat all the ingredients together (except the tortillas).

Place a couple of large spoonfulls of the mixed ingredients into a flat tortilla, and roll it together.

Place filled tortilla into a 9" x 12" casserole pan. Repeat this procedure with the rest of the tortillas, placing them side by side.

Pour a little picante sauce over the casserole and place the 1/2 cup of remaining cheese over the top. Bake for 30 minutes.

Top with dollops of low-fat sour cream.

Garden Street Ratatouille
Yield: 8 servings

Ratatouille is a classic, healthful vegetable stew that originated in France. Overflowing with nutrient-laden carbohydrates, our version makes splendid company fare during the late summer, when veggies are plentiful and reasonably priced.

**1/4 cup olive oil
1 small onion, diced
1 clove garlic, crushed
1 small, unpeeled eggplant, cut into 1/2" cubes
2 small zucchini, cut crosswise into 1/2" slices**

2 celery stalks, cut crosswise into 1/2" slices
1/4 cup diced radish
1 small green bell pepper, cut into 1/2" squares
2 small tomatoes, peeled, seeded, and cut into wedges
1/4 pound mushrooms, cut into quarters
1 tablespoon chopped fresh parsley
1/2 teaspoon dried basil leaves
1/2 teaspoon dried oregano leaves
1/4 teaspoon pepper
1/3 cup slivered almonds

Heat olive oil in a large skillet; add onion and garlic. Saut_ for two to three minutes.

Add eggplant, zucchini, celery, and radish; saut_ for about 5 minutes. Stir in bell pepper, tomatoes, mushrooms, parsley, pepper, and herbs. Simmer, uncovered, for six to eight minutes or until vegetables are tender.

Serve hot.

La Playa Potatoes
Yield: 4 servings

A generous helping of these scalloped potatoes will satisfy the heartiest appetite and provide lots of energy-building carbohydrates. You may want to substitute broccoli or asparagus for the diced carrot.

4 baking potatoes (about 2 pounds total), left unpeeled
1 large carrot, diced
1-1/2 tablespoons butter or margarine
1/8 teaspoon garlic powder
1-1/2 tablespoons whole-wheat flour
1/2 cup low-fat cheddar cheese, grated
2 tablespoons freshly grated Parmesan cheese
1/2 cup thinly sliced onions
   freshly ground black pepper, to taste
1 tablespoon parsley
1 cup shelled peas, steamed briefly
2 cups nonfat or low-fat milk
Additional Parmesan, as desired

Preheat oven to 350° F.

Clean potatoes and cut into 1/8" slices.

Place one-third of the potato slices in a lightly oiled 8" x 8" pan, and sprinkle with one-third of the diced carrot.

Divide the remaining ingredients listed above, except for the peas and milk, in half, and layer them over the potatoes and carrots in the order listed.

Place another one-third of the potato slices and carrots on top, and layer with the remaining halved ingredients plus the peas.

Top with the rest of the potatoes and carrots, and pour the milk over all.

Sprinkle with additional Parmesan and bake for 1-1/2 hours.

Olé Fiesta Salad
Yield: 4-6 servings

The ingredients list for this salad is long, but the preparation is quick and simple. Plus the beans, corn, corn chips, and cheese fulfill your body's requirements for protein, and the v eggies supply you with essential vitamins and minerals.

2 tablespoons olive oil
1-1/2 cooked kidney beans
1 cup cooked brown rice
1/2 cup corn kernels, cooked and cooled
1/4 diced onions
1 garlic clove, minced
1/2 teaspoon chili powder
1/2 teaspoon cumin powder
1/2 teaspoon garlic powder
1/4 pound cheddar cheese, grated
1 head romaine lettuce, torn into bite-size pieces
2 large tomatoes, diced
1 can (4 oz.) diced green chilies (optional)
1/4 pound unsalted, dry-roasted corn chips
  (Note: you can make your own by heating corn tortillas for 10 minutes in a 350° F. oven and then cutting or breaking the crisp tortillas into small pieces.)
  handful alfalfa sprouts
  sour cream, guacamole, and/or ranch dressing (optional)

In a large skillet, place butter or margarine, beans, rice, corn, onions, garlic, and spices. Heat for about seven minutes, and then sprinkle with about 2 tablespoons of the grated cheddar cheese. Cool mixture and set aside.

In a large salad bowl, toss lettuce, tomatoes, chilies, and olives. Mound bean and rice mixture on top. Sprinkle remaining cheese and the corn chips over and around the bean and rice mixture. Spread sprouts around the sides.

Serve on individual salad plates, and pass sour cream, guacamole, and/or ranch dressing as accompaniments.

No-Fuss Tostadas
Yield: 4-6 servings

Feeling a little fatigued? Trying to conserve your energy for the afternoon's activities? Not only will this recipe prevent lunchtime exertion in the kitchen, it will contribute to your energy levels by supplying you with high-quality carbohydrates and protein.

 1 can (16 oz.) vegetarian refried beans or 1 cup cooked pinto beans
 2 cups cooked rice
 6 corn tortillas
 1-1/2 cup shredded low-fat cheddar or Monterey jack cheese
 2 large tomatoes, sliced into wedges
 1 small head iceberg or romaine lettuce, shredded
 3 green onions, finely chopped
 1 ripe avocado, sliced
 1 small can of chopped olives, drained
 Tabasco sauce, to taste
 1/2 cup sour cream (optional)
 guacamole (optional)

Preheat oven to 350° F.

Place corn tortillas on a baking sheet in the oven and bake for 10 minutes or until crisp.

Mound a portion of beans and rice in the center of each crisp tortilla, sprinkle with cheese, and bake for another 10 minutes.

Place tortillas on individual plates, and top with tomatoes, lettuce, onions, avocado, chopped olives, and a dash of Tabasco sauce. If you wish, add a spoonful of guacamole and a dollop of sour cream to each tostada.

Protein-Packed Pocket
Yield: 1 serving

Stash a Protein-Packed Pocket in your lunch sack and see how invigorating a midday meal can be. This sandwich has just the right amount of crunch and zip to perk up your afternoon.

2 ounces tofu, crumbled
1/4 cup diced green bell pepper
1/2 tomato, chopped
1 green onion, chopped
1 tablespoon mayonnaise
1 whole-wheat pocket (pita) bread, cut in half
20 dry-roasted pistachios, chopped
handful alfalfa or bean sprouts

In a medium-sized bowl, mix tofu, vegetables, and mayonnaise.

Stuff the mixture into both halves of the pocket bread, and sprinkle pistachios and sprouts on top.

Serve with an apple and our California Cool Slaw.

Pignoli Pasta Salad
Yield: 4 servings

Whip this tasty salad up tonight while you're doing your dinner dishes, and you'll have a satisfying, energizing lunch to pack in your sack tomorrow. Pignoli—pine nuts—coupled with pasta offer your body the best and most complete protein possible. Of course, pasta is an ideal carbohydrate that fills you up and keeps your blood sugar levels even.

2-1/2 cups spiral (rotelle) pasta, uncooked

1/2 cup olive oil (preferably cold-pressed for best flavor)
1/3 cup vinegar
1 large tomato, chopped
2 green onions, chopped
1/4 cup diced red or green bell pepper
1/4 teaspoon dried basil leaves
1/4 teaspoon Italian herb blend
1/4 teaspoon minced onion flakes
dash black pepper
dash paprika
1/2 cup raisins (optional)
1/2 cup diced cucumber (optional)
4 mushrooms, chopped (optional)
2 tablespoons grated Parmesan cheese (optional)
1/2 cup pignoli (pine nuts) or slivered almonds

Cook pasta al dente according to package directions. Rinse under cold running water.

In a large bowl, combine pasta, vegetables, herbs, spices, and any optional ingredients.

Cover and place in the refrigerator. Let flavors blend for at least two hours or overnight.

Sprinkle pignoli or almonds on top just before serving.

Pizzazzy Pizza Dough
Yield: 6 individual pizzas

When not topped with lots of fat, pizza can make an extremely healthy, soul- and body-satisfying meal. Although this recipe is not exactly quick, the results will invite plenty of compliments and requests for more. In fact, you may want to double the ingredients for this recipe and the filling recipes that follow. Also, consider freezing your homemade pizzas to eat on busy days when you don't have time to cook.

1 cup warm water (about 105° F. or 40° C.)
1 tablespoon (or one package) active dry yeast
1 teaspoon honey
2 tablespoons olive oil
3 cups whole-wheat flour, sifted
1 tablespoon dried Italian herb blend (or use a mixture of dried basil, oregano, and parsley)

Pour warm water into a large glass or ceramic bowl. Sprinkle yeast over the water, add the honey, and stir to dissolve the ingredients. Let yeast mixture stand for 5-10 minutes or until bubbly.

Stir in the oil and one cup of the flour, and beat well. Mix in the herbs and enough of the remaining 2 cups of flour to make a soft dough.

Turn dough out onto a floured board and knead for about five minutes or until dough appears smooth and satiny.

Grease a glass or ceramic bowl, and place dough inside, turning dough over to grease the top. Cover with plastic wrap or a damp dish towel, and place in a warm, draft-free place for about an hour or until the dough has doubled in volume.

In the meantime, preheat oven to 425° F.

Punch down dough to remove air, and then divide dough into six equal parts. On a baking sheet, pat each portion into a 6" circle. Pinch edge to form a rim around each dough circle. Add your desired topping (see recipes that follow), and bake for about 15 minutes or until crust is golden brown and topping is bubbly.

Pizzazzy Pizza Toppings
Yield: enough for six small pizzas

You can top our Pizzazzy Pizza Dough with just about anything that sounds good to you. (But do be careful with the cheese, which can turn an otherwise nutritious pizza into a high-fat food.) Here are recipes for four of our favorite—and healthiest—toppings:

1) Fiesta Combo

olive oil, as needed to brush on pizza crusts
1 can (4 oz.) diced green chilies
4 tomatoes, sliced
2 ripe avocados, sliced (optional)
1/3 cup sliced ripe olives
1/3 cup cooked corn kernels
2 tablespoons chopped green onions
2 tablespoons chopped fresh cilantro (optional)
1 cup shredded low-fat Monterey jack cheese
Pizzazzy Pizza Dough (see previous recipe)

Brush each individual pizza crust with olive oil, and top with chilies, tomatoes, avocados, olives, corn, and green onions. Sprinkle with cilantro and cheese. Bake for about 15 minutes.

2) Shades of the Orient

1/4 cup sesame oil
2 tablespoons minced crystallized ginger
1 tablespoon orange juice
4 tomatoes, sliced
3/4 cup sliced water chestnuts
1/4 cup diced snow peas
2 tablespoons chopped onions
3/4 cup low-fat cheese (your choice)
Pizzazzy Pizza Dough (see previous recipe)

In a large bowl, combine the oil, ginger, and orange juice. Add the tomatoes, water chestnuts, snow peas, and onions. Marinate for at least one hour.

Top individual pizza crusts with tomato mixture. Sprinkle cheese over all, and bake for about 15 minutes.

3) Italiano Classico

1 cup tomato sauce
1 small onion, chopped
1 clove garlic, minced
1/4 cup sliced mushrooms
1/4 cup sliced ripe olives (optional)
1/4 cup diced green bell pepper
2 tablespoons pignoli (pine nuts)
1 tablespoon chopped fresh parsley
1/4 cup part-skim mozzarella cheese
1/4 cup low-fat Monterey jack cheese
1/4 cup freshly grated Parmesan cheese
Pizzazzy Pizza Dough (see previous recipe)

Spread tomato sauce on individual pizza crusts. Distribute onion, garlic, mushrooms, olives, bell pepper, pignoli, and parsley among the six crusts. Top with the cheeses and bake for about 15 minutes.

4) Santa Barbara Nouvelle

1/3 cup olive oil
1 tablespoon fresh, chopped tarragon
2 tomatoes, sliced
1/2 cup chopped walnuts (optional)
1/2 cup diced pineapple
1/4 cup raisins
3 ounces thinly sliced goat cheese
1/4 cup freshly grated Parmesan cheese
Pizzazzy Pizza Dough (see previous recipe)

In a medium-sized bowl, combine olive oil, tarragon, and tomatoes, and marinate at room temperature for at least one hour. (Refrigerate if you choose to marinate the tomatoes for more than a couple of hours.)

Spread individual pizza crusts with tomato mixture, walnuts, pineapple raisins, and goat cheese. Sprinkle with Parmesan and bake for about 15 minutes.

Ranch-Style Fettucine
Yield: 3 servings

Serve your favorite ranch hand a plate of hot fettucine tossed with fresh vegetables. Pasta is a super-powered, gradually digested carbohydrate that gives the body all the right nutrients for a long afternoon's chores.

1/4 cup butter or margarine
1 medium zucchini, cut into matchstick-sized pieces
1 carrot, cut into matchstick-sized pieces
6 mushrooms, sliced
1/4 cup sliced green onions
1 clove garlic, minced
1/2 teaspoon dried basil leaves
1/8 teaspoon freshly ground black pepper
dash dried parsley flakes
1/2 cup green peas, cooked
12 oz. uncooked fettucine
1/4 cup freshly grated Parmesan cheese

Melt butter or margarine in a medium skillet over medium heat. Add zucchini and carrot, and saut_ until nearly tender. Stir in mushrooms, onions, garlic, basil, pepper, and parsley flakes; cook for two minutes. Add peas and cook only until the peas are hot.

In the meantime, cook fettucine al dente according to package directions. Drain and place in a large bowl.

Gently toss fettucine with cooked vegetables and grated Parmesan. Serve immediately.

La Cumbre Salad
Yield: 4 servings

La Cumbre, Spanish for "the peak," is a summit in the nearby Santa Ynez mountain range that borders Santa Barbara and makes the area a coastal oasis. We like to call this salad "La Cumbre" because it offers a kind of peak eating experience: it fills us up, satisfies our taste buds, and looks spectacular. Plus it's great to share with friends.

1/4 head romaine lettuce, torn into bite-size pieces
1/4 head red leaf lettuce, torn into bite-size pieces
1/4 head green cabbage, shredded
1/2 cucumber, sliced crosswise
1 tomato, chopped
5 asparagus tips, steamed and chopped
8 snow peas, diced
1/4 diced bell pepper
1/4 cup sliced mushrooms
1/2 cup cubed Monterey jack cheese (optional)
1/2 cup chopped walnuts (optional)
1/2 cup diced dried papaya (optional)
1/2 cup alfalfa sprouts (optional)
1/2 cup grated carrot

In a large salad bowl, toss all the ingredients listed above except the grated carrot. Use the latter as a garnish.

Serve with Sass Splash, Zesty Bleu Cheese Dressing, or one of our other dressings.

Irresistible Lasagna Roll-ups
Yield: 3-6 servings

You may find this easily assembled, delectable dish so popular that you'll decide to double it. The combination of pasta, spinach, tomato sauce, and cottage cheese creates a perfectly rounded entrée that provides most essential nutrients.

6 plain or spinach lasagna noodles, cooked

Filling

2-1/2 cups finely chopped spinach
1 cup low-fat cottage cheese (for a richer, smoother filling, use
1/2 cup part-skim ricotta cheese and 1/2 cup low-fat cottage cheese)
1/4 cup freshly grated Parmesan cheese
1 egg, beaten (optional)
1/2 teaspoon nutmeg
1/2 teaspoon fennel seed

Sauce

3 cups (approximately) tomato sauce
1 teaspoon garlic powder
1 teaspoon onion powder

Preheat oven to 350° F.

To make filling, combine all ingredients in a medium-sized bowl and mix well.

To make sauce, combine tomato sauce with garlic and onion powders.

Spread each cooked noodle evenly with the filling, and then roll up noodles carefully. Place on end in a lightly greased baking dish or casserole. Cover with sauce and bake for about 20 minutes or until roll-ups are heated through and sauce is bubbly.

Sisquoc Squash
Yield: 3 servings

This heart-and hearth-warming entrée combines the high-quality carbohydrates and vitamins of acorn squash with the protein of grains, walnuts, wheat germ, and cheese.

1-1/2 cups cooked bulgur or wild rice
3/4 cup wheat germ
1 medium onion, finely chopped
2 tablespoons chopped walnuts
2 egg whites, slightly beaten
2 teaspoons chopped fresh parsley
1/2 teaspoon dried sage
1/4 teaspoon ground black pepper
3 acorn squash, cut in half and seeds removed
1/2 cup grated Monterey jack cheese (optional)

Preheat oven to 350° F.

In a medium-sized bowl, combine all ingredients except squash and cheese. Loosely pack mixture in six squash halves. Sprinkle with cheese, if desired.

Lightly oil a pan. Place stuffed squash in pan and cover loosely with aluminum foil. Bake for one hour or until squash is tender.

Franceschi Stuffed Peppers
Yield: 2 servings

Need a boost of vitamin C? Tired of relying on orange juice for your daily dose? Try eating low-calorie bell peppers, which also contain lots of potassium and vitamin A. Stuff these sweet v eggies with brown rice and other goodies, bake them for just a few minutes, and you've got a nutritious pepper-upper.

2 green or red bell peppers
1 cup cooked brown rice
1/2 cup crumbled tofu or 1/2 cup low-fat cottage cheese
8 walnuts, diced (optional)
1 egg, beaten (optional)

1 tablespoon toasted wheat germ
1 tablespoon freshly grated Parmesan cheese (optional)
1 tablespoon tamari
1 clove garlic, minced
1 teaspoon minced onion
1 teaspoon dried parsley flakes
1/2 teaspoon dried oregano
1/2 teaspoon dried rosemary
dash cayenne pepper
dash paprika

Preheat oven to 350° F.
Slice tops off peppers and scoop out seeds.
In a medium-sized bowl, blend all ingredients except Parmesan cheese and paprika.
Stuff peppers with the mixture; sprinkle cheese and paprika on top.
Place peppers upright in a lightly oiled casserole and bake for 20 minutes or until tops are crisp.

Tucker's Grove Loaf
Yield: 6 servings

What's far healthier than meatloaf but just as easy to make and eat? A vegetarian rice, bean, and sunflower loaf, naturally. Try topping this slightly crunchy main dish with a little unsweetened ketchup.

3 cups cooked brown rice
1-1/2 cups diced string beans
1 cup chopped onion
1/2 cup toasted sunflower seeds
1/2 cup grated carrots
1/4 cup minced fresh parsley
1/4 cup sunflower or safflower oil
1 clove garlic, minced
2 tablespoons whole-wheat flour
2 tablespoons water
1/2 teaspoon each dried thyme, basil, oregano, and rosemary
2 eggs, beaten (optional)

Preheat oven to 350° F.

Mix ingredients thoroughly and place in a large, lightly oiled loaf pan. Cover pan with aluminum foil so that the flavors and moisture stay in.

Bake for about 45 minutes or until top appears golden.

Sandpiper Sunburgers
Yield: 6 patties

These chewy, high-fiber, high-iron "burgers' provide a quick, healthy alternative to greasy hamburgers. While your sunburgers bake, toss a lightly seasoned green salad or mix up small fruit-and-yogurt shakes to round out your repast.

1-1/2 cups ground sunflower seeds (dry-roasted or raw, shells removed) or 1 cup ground sunflower seeds and 1/2 cup
   ground dry-roasted peanuts
1/2 cup grated carrots
1/2 cup finely chopped celery
6 tablespoons minced onion
1/4 cup green bell pepper, diced
2 eggs, beaten
2 tablespoons minced parsley
2 tablespoons tamari
2 tablespoons brewer's yeast
1 teaspoon dried basil
1 teaspoon garlic powder
whole-grain buns

Preheat oven to 350° F.

In a large bowl, combine the first 11 ingredients. Drop mixture by large spoonfuls onto a lightly oiled baking sheet, and then form into patties.

Bake patties for 20 minutes on one side, flip them, and bake for an additional 10 to 15 minutes or until both sides are nicely browned.

Serve on buns, and accompany with all your favorite condiments.

Invigorating Tofu-Salad Sandwich
Yield: 2 sandwiches

What a great alternative to cholesterol-heavy egg salad! The dill pickle adds just the right tartness to the creamy tofu, the soybean product that contains lots of protein but absolutely no cholesterol.

4 ounces firm tofu, drained
1 medium dill pickle, chopped (about 2 tablespoons)
1 stalk celery, chopped finely
1 tablespoon soy mayonnaise
1/2 teaspoon prepared mustard
1/4 teaspoon minced onion
1/4 teaspoon turmeric
1/2 cucumber, sliced thinly
4 slices whole-grain bread

In a medium-sized bowl, crumble the tofu into small pieces with a fork. Add the pickle, celery, soy mayonnaise, mustard, onion, and turmeric. Mix well.
Spread on bread slices and top with cucumber slices.

Zucchini á la Zucker
Yield: 6 servings

A sort of lasagna without the noodles, this perfectly rounded meal-in-a-pan offers your body necessary carbohydrates, protein, vitamins, and minerals.

4 medium zucchini, unpeeled
1 onion, chopped
1/2 pound tofu, crumbled
1/2 cup sliced mushrooms
1/2 cup chopped almonds
2 cans (8 oz. each) tomato sauce
1 can (6 oz.) tomato paste
1/2 cup water
1 tablespoon chopped fresh parsley
1/2 teaspoon dried oregano
1/4 teaspoon ground black pepper

1 egg
2 cups low-fat cottage cheese
8oz. sliced mozzarella cheese
1/2 cup grated Parmesan cheese (about 1-1/2 oz.)

Steam or boil whole zucchini until barely tender, about 10 minutes. Drain and cut lengthwise into 1/4" slices. Set aside.

In a large skillet, saut_ onion, tofu, mushrooms, and onions until browned. Add tomato sauce, tomato paste, water, herbs, and pepper. Cover and simmer for 35 minutes.

Preheat oven to 350° F.

In a small bowl, beat egg and mix in cottage cheese; set aside.

Spread one-third of the cooked tomato sauce on the bottom of a 13" x 9" baking pan. Arrange one-third of the sliced, cooked zucchini on top of the sauce. Top with one-third of the egg and cottage cheese mixture and one-third of the mozzarella cheese slices. Repeat this layering procedure two more times.

Sprinkle the top with grated Parmesan cheese, and bake 40 to 45 minutes or until bubbly.

Serve hot.

Spaghetti Isla Vista
Yield: 1 serving

This is the quickest spaghetti dish we know, so we named it for the area in which most of Santa Barbara's time-and health-conscious college students live. The hot noodles help to steam the fresh veggies just a tad.

2-4 ounces dry whole-wheat spaghetti
1/2 zucchini, grated
1/2 tomato, diced
1/2 stalk celery, diced
2 small mushrooms, sliced
1 tablespoon chopped onion
1 teaspoon garlic powder
1 teaspoon dried basil leaves
1 teaspoon butter or margarine
1 tablespoon freshly grated Parmesan cheese

Cook spaghetti al dente according to package directions. Drain.

Meanwhile, in a medium-sized bowl, place zucchini, tomato slices, celery, mushrooms, onion, garlic powder, and basil. Add hot noodles and toss gently.

Transfer spaghetti to a plate and top with butter or margarine and Parmesan cheese. Serve.

Country-Club Asparagus
Yield: 4 servings

This sensational springtime dish is worthy of the finest company. Fresh asparagus spears give your body a good supply of niacin, a B-complex vitamin that assists digestion, as well as vitamins A and C.

2 pounds fresh asparagus
3 tablespoons butter or margarine or 1/4 cup olive oil
2 teaspoons lemon juice
1 teaspoon parsley
2/3 cup dry-roasted cashew pieces

Steam asparagus just until tender.

In a saucepan, melt butter or margarine over low heat; add lemon juice and parsley. Simmer for a couple of minutes.

Pour butter or margarine over hot asparagus, and sprinkle cashews on top. Serve immediately.

Speedy Stuffed tomatoes
Yield: 3-6 servings

This gourmet, eye-catching vegetable dish tastes particularly wonderful with our Sandpiper Sunburgers.

3 large tomatoes, cut in halves
1/4 cup soft, whole-wheat bread crumbs
2 tablespoons rasins (optional)
1 tablespoon butter or margarine, melted
1/2 teaspoon dried basil leaves
1/8 teaspoon ground black pepper
1/2 cup (2 oz.) shredded Monterey jack cheese
1 tablespoon chopped fresh parsley

Preheat oven to 375°.

Scoop the pulp out of each tomato half, leaving a shell about 1/2" thick. Chop pulp; set aside.

In a medium-sized bowl, mix bread crumbs, raisins, melted butter or margarine, dried basil, and pepper. Stir in shredded cheese and chopped tomato pulp.

Spoon bread crumb mixture into tomato halves, and place each half, stuffed side up, in a lightly greased casserole or Pyrex dish.

Cover and bake for about 15 minutes. or until the cheese melts.

Sprinkle with parsley, and serve immediately.

Tomatoes Montecito
Yield: 4 servings

Although these stuffed tomatoes will have your fellow diners imagining that you spent all afternoon in the kitchen, this veggie dish only requires a bit of chopping, dicing, and saut_eing. The tomatoes' impressive appearance also belies their high nutritional value. But never mind: simply enjoy the oohs and ahhs; you and your body know the truth.

4 large tomatoes
2 tablespoons olive oil
1 onion, diced
1 stalk celery, chopped
1 green bell pepper, seeded and diced
1 cup corn kernels
1/2 cup chopped mushrooms
1 clove garlic, minced
1/4 cup grated low-fat Monterey jack or cheddar cheese
1/4 cup whole-grain bread crumbs or 1/4 cup
   toasted wheat germ

Preheat oven to 350° F.

Cut off tops of tomatoes and remove pulp with a teaspoon, leaving shells about 1/2" thick.

In a large skillet, heat oil and saut_ onion, celery, bell pepper, corn, mushrooms, and garlic until tender. Transfer to a large bowl.

To the warm vegetables add half the cheese and enough bread crumbs or wheat germ to hold the mixture together.

Stuff tomatoes with vegetable mixture and place tomatoes in a lightly greased baking pan or casserole. Sprinkle with remaining cheese and bread crumbs, and bake for 15 minutes or until cheese has melted and tops are golden.

Short-Order Sweet Potatoes
Yield: 4 servings

Here's a quick and appetizing way to cook sweet potatoes, a vegetable that is particularly rich in vitamin A, which is a nutrient that helps you battle infections and keeps your skin looking healthy.

2 tablespoons butter or margarine
2 pounds slender sweet potatoes, peeled
  and cut crosswise into 1/4" slices
1 large onion, chopped
2 large green bell peppers, diced
1-1/2 tablespoons sesame seeds
  tamari, to taste
1/4 cup chopped pe cans (optional)

In a large skillet, melt butter or margarine and saut_ sweet potato slices and chopped onion for about 15 minutes.

Add remaining ingredients and sauté for an additional 10 to 15 minutes or until vegetables are tender. Stir in pecans. Serve hot.

Cabana Curried Rice
Yield: 4-6 servings

Brown rice mixed with fresh veggies offers active people the fiber, protein, and carbohydrates their bodies need to function at maximum capacity; a touch of curry makes this body-building grain and vegetable dish even more palatable. If you wish, you may use about three cups of already cooked, leftover brown rice.

1-1/2 cups uncooked brown rice
3 cups water
1 tablespoon oil
1/2 medium zucchini, shredded
1/2 cup chopped onion
1/2 cup chopped green pepper
1 clove garlic, minced
1/2 cup corn kernels
1/2 cup raisins
1/4 cup sliced olives
1/4 teaspoon curry powder or more, to taste

Cook rice in 3 cups of water for 45 minutes or until done. Leave in pan and set aside.

In a medium skillet, heat oil and sauté zucchini, onion, bell pepper, and garlic until soft. Add corn, raisins, olives, curry powder, and water. Simmer 10 minutes.

Add onion mixture to rice, cover, and cook for and additional 15 minutes. (You may wish to add two tablespoons of water before cooking so that the rice doesn't stick to the pan.) Serve hot.

Alamar Eggplant Medley
Yield: 2 servings

Light and savory, this vegetable-and-herb combo offers good dietary fiber as well as good flavor.

1 small eggplant
1 medium zucchini
1 teaspoon tamari
2 tablespoons olive oil
1 tablespoon chopped fresh chives
1 tablespoon chopped fresh parsley
1/2 teaspoon oregano
1/4 teaspoon dried basil leaves
1/4 teaspoon dried marjoram leaves
    grated Parmesan or slivered almonds (optional)

Shred unpeeled eggplant and zucchini in a food processor

or on a hand-held grater. Sprinkle with tamari and toss to mix.

Place shredded eggplant and zucchini in a colander over a bowl or pie plate. Let drain for one-half hour; squeeze out excess water.

In a medium-sized skillet, heat olive oil. Add shredded eggplant and zucchini, and sauté for five or six minutes or until nearly tender.

Add herbs, and cover and cook for one minute.

Sprinkle with Parmesan or almonds, if desired. Serve hot.

Padaro Lane Potatoes
Yield: 6 servings

We've named this rich-tasting potato dish after a lane on which some rich and famous Santa Barbarans live. The flavorful figs we include here are an excellent source of dietary fiber.

1/3 cup butter or margarine, melted
1 tablespoon chopped fresh chives
1 tablespoon chopped fresh parsley
1/4 teaspoon fines herbes (a French herb blend)
1/8 teaspoon paprika
1/8 teaspoon ground black pepper
6 medium baking potatoes
1/2 cup diced dried figs
1/4 cup diced tomatoes
1/3 cup (about 1 oz.) freshly grated Parmesan cheese

Preheat oven to 425° F.

In a small bowl, combine melted butter or margarine, chives, parsley, fines herbes, paprika, and pepper; set aside.

Scrub each potato and slice it crosswise at 1/4" intervals, cutting about halfway through the potato. Be careful not to slice completely through the potato.

Brush potatoes with butter or margarine mixture. Wrap each potato in aluminum foil and place all six in a shallow baking pan.

Bake for 30 minutes or until nearly tender.

Fold back foil to expose the top of each potato. Scoop out

the inside of each potato and mash. Combine the mashed potatoes with the figs and tomatoes, and stuff the mixture into the potato jackets. Sprinkle with Parmesan and return the stuffed potatoes to the oven for 10 minutes or tops are golden. Serve hot.

Millet San Marcos
Yield: 3-4 servings

This recipe enhances the naturally nutty taste of millet, a nourishing grain that is high in protein, B vitamins and a number of minerals.

2 cups water
1 cup millet
4 tablespoons olive oil
1 small onion, minced
1/2 red bell pepper, diced
2 cloves garlic, minced
1/4 cup sliced mushrooms
1-1/2 teaspoons chopped fresh parsley
1/2 teaspoon dried thyme leaves
1/2 teaspoon dried basil leaves
1/2 teaspoon dried tarragon leaves
1/2 teaspoon herb blend
pinch ground black pepper
1/4 cup sesame seeds

Boil water in a medium-sized saucepan, and add millet. Simmer for 15 minutes.

Add remaining ingredients and cook for an additional 10 minutes. Stir in sesame seeds and serve hot.

Lively, Lemony Beans
Yield: 4 servings

For a nutritious, light supper, accompany this delectable cheese-and-bean dish with whole-grain bread and a refreshing drink.

1 pound fresh green beans, steamed
1/3 cup butter or margarine, melted
2 large cloves garlic, minced
1 teaspoon dried thyme leaves
1 teaspoon dried basil leaves
3/4 teaspoon dried oregano leaves
dash ground black pepper, or to taste
5 tablespoons or more fresh lemon juice
1/2 cup freshly grated Parmesan cheese or
  1/2 cup shredded low-fat Monterey jack cheese

Preheat oven to 375° F.

Spread string beans in a 2-1/2 quart baking dish.

Combine butter or margarine with garlic, herbs, pepper, and lemon juice. Add mixture to beans and stir well. Sprinkle with cheese.

Bake for 15 to 20 minutes or until beans are quite hot and cheese is melted.

Variation: Use asparagus or cauliflower in place of beans.

Skinny Spuds
Yield: 4-6 servings

We adore mashed potatoes, so we devised this fat-free recipe for fluffy, rich-tasting "spuds."

6 medium potatoes
1-1/2 cups nonfat milk
1 tablespoon tamari
1 tablespoon fresh lemon juice
1 teaspoon dried parsley flakes
dash pepper

Scrub potatoes, or peel them, if desired. Cube and boil until tender. Drain and mash well, adding milk, tamari, lemon juice, parsley, and pepper.

Serve piping hot.

Note: A sprinkling (about 4 tablespoons) of dry-roasted sunflower seeds adds extra protein and flavor.

Polo Field Paté
Yield: 4-6 servings

Take this appetizing mushroom spread in your picnic basket to the next polo match or outdoor concert. Then enjoy your impressive, gourmet paté on crackers, whole-grain rolls, or sourdough slices.

1 pound fresh mushrooms, sliced
1 small onion, sliced
1 clove garlic, minced
3 tablespoons water
1/2 cup slivered almonds, toasted
1 tablespoon oil
1 teaspoon tamari
1/4 teaspoon dried thyme leaves
1 tablespoon chopped fresh parsley

Steam until tender the mushrooms, onions, and garlic in the 3 tablespoons of water. Remove from heat, drain, and reserve the liquid.

Coarsely chop the toasted almonds in blender or food processor; remove one tablespoon and set aside. Continue chopping remaining nuts, slowly adding oil until mixture is well blended.

To the almonds in the blender add tamari, thyme, and mushrooms, and blend thoroughly. If the mixture looks dry, add the reserved mushroom liquid.

Remove from blender and stir in the reserved tablespoon of almonds. Mold into a loaf or a ball on an attractive serving dish, and sprinkle with chopped parsley.

Palm Park Peas
Yield: 3-4 servings

This colorful combination of lettuce and peas has French origins. The vegetables braise in their own juices, creating a kind of hot salad that complements pasta, potatoes, or grain dishes beautifully.

2 teaspoons butter or margarine
10-12 lettuce or cabbage leaves, shredded into 1/4" strips
3 cups shelled fresh or frozen peas
1/2 red bell pepper, diced
1/4 cup finely chopped onion
1/4 cup diced carrots
1 clove garlic, minced
1/4 cup water
1/4 teaspoon ground black pepper

In a saucepan, melt the butter or margarine. Add lettuce and top with peas, bell pepper, onion, carrots, and garlic.
Cover tightly and cook over medium heat or until peas are tender. Sprinkle with pepper and serve.

Ballard Bean Salad
Yield: 2 servings

Here's another simple salad that travels well. For a deliciously complete meal, accompany this piquant salad with brown rice.

1/2 cup raw string beans, cut into bite-size pieces
1/4 cup cooked kidney beans
1/4 cup diced cucumber
1 stalk celery, chopped
1 green onion, chopped
1 clove garlic, minced
dash dried basil leaves
dash dried parsley flakes
1/2 cup apple-cider vinegar
2 tablespoons olive oil

Combine all ingredients and chill for a few hours or overnight.

Potato Crisps
Yield: 4 servings

Who can resist French fries? We can! Especially when we know that we can prepare a healthy version that really tastes like potatoes and not just fat.

4 medium potatoes
1 tablespoon sesame or corn oil
paprika, to taste

Preheat oven to 450° F.
Scrub potatoes, cut into strips about 1/2" thick. As you are cutting, place potato strips in a bowl of ice water to keep them from browning. Drain and pat strips dry with a paper towel.
Return potato strips to bowl, and sprinkle with oil. Mix with hands to distribute oil evenly over potatoes.
Spread strips on a large (jell-roll) baking pan, and bake until they are golden brown and tender, about 30 to 40 minutes, stirring and turning the potatoes frequently.
Sprinkle generously with paprika and serve.

Note: Our Potato Crisps taste wonderful served with sugar-free ketchup or low-calorie sour cream.

Daniel's Meal-in-a-Muffin
Yield: 2 dozen

Warm, savory baked goods. Nothing else tastes or smells more appetizing at the end of a long day, so we're supplying you with a recipe for quick muffins that will serve as a light entrée or a late-night snack. In fact, you can freeze these and reheat them when you want a dinner-on-the-run.

1 lb. fresh spinach, washed and chopped or
1-10 oz. package   frozen spinach, thawed and drained
1 cup w/w pastry flour
1/2 cup corn meal
1/3 cup olive oil
1/3 cup shredded low-fat Monterey jack cheese
1/4 cup unsweetened pineapple juice concentrate
2 green onions, chopped
2 eggs, beaten
1 teaspoon ground nutmeg
1 teaspoon dried parsley flakes

Preheat oven to 350° F.
In a large bowl, mix all ingredients just until moistened.
(Do you need to cook the spinach first?)
    Spoon into two lightly oiled muffin tins. Bake for about 25 minutes or until muffins are golden.

Cuyama carrots
Yield: 4 servings

Cuyama is a remote town just north of our Sierra Madre Mountains that boasts fields filled with sweet carrots. See if you can wrangle up some freshly harvested carrots, and try them with the sweet-and-sour sauce in this recipe. The sauce will satisfy your late-afternoon sweet tooth; the carrots' vitamin A will encourage the healthy growth of your bones, skin, and hair.

6 medium carrots
2 tablespoons butter or margarine
25 seedless green grapes, cut in half
1/2 cup diced pineapple with juice
2 tablespoons honey
1 tablespoon tamari
1/2 teaspoon grated orange peel

Cut carrots diagonally into 1/4" slices.
    Melt butter or margarine in a medium-sized skillet. Add carrot slices and sauté for about two minutes.

Add grapes, pineapple, honey, tamari, and orange peel. Cover and simmer 10 to 15 minutes or until carrots are tender. Serve hot.

Tabouli Take-out
Yield: 4 servings

Have a hankering for a crunchy take-out salad? Then why not make your own? If you plan a head, this great grain salad can await you when you come home from work. Here is our version of tabouli, a classic Mideastern dish made from bulgur, which is a type of cracked wheat.

3-1/2 cups boiling water
2 cups dry bulgur wheat
1-1/2 cups lemon juice
1/8 cup sunflower or safflower oil
2-1/2 cups (packed) finely chopped
  parsley (about 4 large bunches)
3 tomatoes, finely diced
1 celery stalk, chopped
3/4 cup chopped green onions, including tops
1/2 cup chopped, peeled jécama
1 tablespoon dried mint leaves, or fresh mint, to taste
1 tablespoon tamari
1-1/2 teaspoons garlic powder
1 teaspoon ground black pepper

In a large bowl, combine boiling water and bulgur. Allow bulgur to soak for at least one hour.

Mix in remaining ingredients and chill for at least two hours.

Beet-It Salad
Yield: 4-6 servings

This festive-looking dish, which you can make in advance, tastes both sweet and tangy. It offers energetic bodies a good dose of potassium, the nutrient that helps lower blood pressure naturally.

1/2 cup mayonnaise
1/3 cup plain nonfat or low-fat yogurt
4 cups diced cooked beets
1/2 cup diced red bell pepper
1/2 cucumber, diced
3 radishes, diced
2 tablespoons finely chopped green onions or fresh chives
2 tablespoons lemon juice
1 tablespoon chopped fresh parsley

In a large bowl, combine mayonnaise and yogurt. Mix in remaining ingredients, and add more lemon juice according to your taste.
Chill until ready to serve.

El Capitan Potato Salad
Yield: 4-6 servings

This is the kind of crunchy, munchy entrée salad we love to take to the beach. It's simple and easy to eat, and it's particularly satisfying after a taxing game of Frisbee or volleyball. Plus the potatoes' complex carbohydrates and the cashews' iron prevent fatigue and replenish our dwindling energy supplies.

3/4 pound red "new" potatoes, cooked and cubed
3/4 cup chopped dry-roasted cashews
3/4 celery stalk, diced
1/2 cucumber, diced
1/4 cup chopped green onions
1/4 cup diced red apple
2/3 cup soy mayonnaise
1/2 cup apple-cider vinegar

In a large bowl, mix vegetables, apple, and cashews. Combine vinegar and mayonnaise, and pour over potato mixture. Toss well and chill.

Seaside Caesar Salad
Yield: 4 servings

This recipe makes us think of romantic sunset dinners. Why? Because many elegant restaurants serve a version of this classic, garlicky salad. Serve your Caesar Salad with sparkling cider and slices of sourdough, and turn a light meal into an intimate gathering.

1/4 cup olive oil
1 clove garlic, crushed
3/4 cup sourdough bread cubes (about 1/2" each)
2 eggs
1 head romaine lettuce
2 tablespoons fresh lemon juice
1 tomato, chopped
1/3 cup soy baco-bits
1/4 cup (about 3/4 oz.) grated Parmesan cheese
1/8 teaspoon pepper

In a small cup, combine olive oil and garlic. Let stand 2 hours, if possible.

Make croutons by browning bread cubes in a 350° F. oven for 20 minutes or until crisp. Set aside to cool.

In a small saucepan, bring a small amount of water to a boil. Gently place the eggs (still in their shells) in the boiling water; leave for one minute. Remove from boiling water and immediately pour cold water over egg. Set egg aside.

Place oil and garlic mixture in a large bowl. Tear romaine into bite-sized pieces and add to bowl. Toss.

Break egg over lettuce, and toss to coat leaves.

Add lemon juice; toss.

Add tomatoes and soy bits; toss.

Add Parmesan and pepper; toss again.

Top with croutons. Serve immediately.

California Cool Slaw
Yield: 3 servings

The dressings on most commercial slaws contain far too

much fat, so we've devised a dressing that's cool, sweet, and good for you. The raw cabbage and grated carrot in this crunchy slaw provide fabulous fiber and lots of vitamin C.

2-1/2 cups shredded green cabbage (or half green and half red cabbage)
1 medium carrot, grated
1/4 cup mayonnaise
1 tablespoon lemon juice
1 tablespoon plain nonfat or low-fat yogurt
1 tablespoon honey
1 tablespoon chopped onion
1 tablespoon raisins
1 tablespoon dry-roasted sunflower seeds, toasted
1 tablespoon diced pineapple or 1/4 cup diced red bell   pepper (optional)
dash pepper

In a medium-sized bowl, combine all ingredients. Refrigerate for several hours or longer.

San Roque Salad
Yield: 6 servings

Suitable for a party, this exotic cole slaw boasts iron-rich dates and naturally sweet coconut.

4 cups (about one small head) shredded green cabbage
1 can (8 oz.) crushed pineapple, drained
1/2 cup chopped dates
1/4 cup chopped celery
1/2 cup dairy sour cream
1 tablespoon honey
1 teaspoon lime juice
1 teaspoon finely chopped crystallized ginger
1/4 cup unsweetened flaked coconut

In a large salad bowl, combine cabbage, pineapple, dates, and celery.

In a small bowl, mix sour cream, honey, lime juice, and ginger. Pour over cabbage mixture; toss lightly.

Sprinkle coconut over slaw. Serve.

Cucumbers Asiana
Yield: 4 servings

This easy-to-make salad accompanies Chinese or Japanese entrées beautifully. You may want to use English hothouse cucumbers, the long, skinny variety that contains fewer seeds but more flavor than the average, garden-grown varieties.

2 cups cucumbers sliced crosswise and paper-thin
20 snow peas
1/4 cup sliced mushrooms
1/2 cup apple-cider vinegar
1 tablespoon honey
1 tablespoon low-sodium soy sauce
1 tablespoon sesame oil
tomato slices for garnish
dried dill weed

Combine all the ingredients except the tomato slices. Toss well and chill for at least two hours. Garnish with tomato slices and sprinkle with dill weed.

Variation: Substitute asparagus for cucumber. To do so, cook 15 to 20 asparagus spears for five minutes or just until tender. Cut spears into 2" pieces and combine with ingredients listed above. Chill.

Quick Cuke Salad
Yield: 4-6 servings

Hot and cool at the same time, this spicy salad complements our Tucker's Grove Loaf or Sandpiper Sunburgers. When accompanied by rice or bread, this light salad can also serve as a quick, complete-protein supper. You'll like the zinginess of cumin and onion coupled with the coolness of cucumber chunks and dairy dressing.

1/2 cup low-fat cottage cheese
1/2 cup plain nonfat or low-fat yogurt
1 teaspoon cumin

1 medium cucumber, chopped
1 small onion, finely chopped
1 tomato, chopped
1 stalk celery, finely chopped
1 tablespoon chopped parsley
dash nutmeg

Blend cottage cheese and yogurt in a blender until smooth. Add cumin.

In a salad bowl, combine vegetables. Pour dressing over and toss.

Refrigerate for at least one half hour before serving.

Devra's Mushroom Salad
Yield: 3 servings

Light and elegant—but easy to assemble—this delicately seasoned salad will please your most discriminating guest. Plus the low-calorie mushrooms contain potassium and niacin, nutrients essential for the healthy functioning of your brain and nervous system.

1/3 cup olive oil
3 tablespoons apple-cider vinegar
1 tablespoon lemon juice
2 tablespoons minced fresh watercress
1 tablespoon minced fresh chives
1 tablespoon minced pimiento
1 teaspoon Dijon-style mustard
1/4 teaspoon dried chervil leaves, crushed
1/4 teaspoon ground black pepper
1/2 pound fresh mushrooms, thinly sliced
1/2 cup diced tomato
red leaf lettuce leaves
1 tablespoon sesame seeds

In a small bowl, mix olive oil, vinegar, lemon juice, watercress, chives, pimiento, mustard, chervil, and pepper.

In a medium-sized bowl, place mushrooms and tomatoes. Add olive oil dressing and and toss lightly.

Line a salad bowl with lettuce leaves. Mound mushroom mixture on lettuce, and sprinkle with sesame seeds. Serve immediately.

Festival Greek Salad
Yield: 4 servings

Every August, the local Greek Orthodox Church hosts a marvelous Greek festival at Oak Park. This crunchy salad, a complete meal in itself, reminds us of that festival.

Note: Made from sheep's or goat's milk, feta cheese has less fat but more salt than cow's milk cheese. To eliminate some of the salt, soak your block of feta in cold water while you prepare the rest of the salad. Drain and crumble the feta just before you're ready to add it to the salad.

1/2 head romaine lettuce, torn into bite-size pieces
1/2 small cauliflower, separated into flowerets
1/2 large green bell pepper, diced
1 carrot, grated
1 medium tomato, chopped
1/2 can (or about 3 ounces) sliced black olives, drained
1/4 pound feta cheese, crumbled
1 clove garlic, minced
1 teaspoon dried basil leaves
3/4 cup plain nonfat or low-fat yogurt
2 tablespoons mayonnaise
1 tablespoon olive oil
1 tablespoon freshly squeezed lemon juice
dash pepper

In a medium-sized bowl, combine vegetables, tomato, olives, cheese, garlic, and basil.
In a small bowl, mix garlic, yogurt, mayonnaise, olive oil, and lemon juice. Pour over vegetable mixture and toss.
Season with black pepper and chill before serving.

Healthy Harvest Salad
Yield: 4-6 servings

A nice alternative to the ubiquitous green salad, this gorgeous combination of golden fruits looks terrific on a festive holiday table. In addition, this salad gives diners tons of vitamins A and C, nutrients that help people look and feel festive.

1 head romaine lettuce or curly endive
2 grapefruits, sectioned and seeded
2 avocados, peeled and sliced
2 oranges, sectioned and seeded
2 soft, ripe persimmons, peeled and sliced (optional)
1/3 cup sesame-seed oil
3 tablespoons lemon juice
1 teaspoon honey
1/2 teaspoon Dijon mustard or dry mustard
2 tablespoons shelled sunflower seeds

Arrange romaine or endive leaves on a large serving plate. Top the greens with alternating layers of grapefruit sections, orange sections, avocado slices, and persimmon slices.

In a small bowl, combine oil, lemon juice, honey, and mustard. Drizzle this dressing over fruit.

Sprinkle fruit with sunflower seeds, and serve the salad immediately.

Lentil Salad Lobero
Yield: 4 servings

Quick and easy to cook, lentils are the basis for this unique salad, which makes a welcome side dish at picnics and potlucks. You can combine all the ingredients, except the greens and tomatoes, a head of time, and then refrigerate or freeze the mixture until you need to assemble the salad.

1-1/2 cups cooked lentils
1/3 cup olive oil
1/2 cup apple-cider vinegar
1/2 teaspoon Tabasco sauce
2 cups chopped celery
1 carrot, diced
1/2 cup chopped onion
2 cloves garlic, minced
1 head red leaf lettuce, washed and chilled
2 tomatoes, cut into wedges
1/4 cup diced pecans (optional)

As soon as you have cooked the lentils, place them in a medium-sized bowl and add oil, vinegar, and Tabasco sauce. Mix well and cool.

Add celery, carrot, onion, and garlic. Chill for several hours.

Turn lentil mixture into a bowl lined with cold lettuce leaves or onto individual serving plates lined with lettuce.

Garnish with tomato wedges and pecans.

Oriental Delight
Yield: 6-8 servings

Accompanied by bread, noodles, or additional rice, this crispy, tangy salad makes a light but filling meal. Napa cabbage (also called Chinese cabbage) is becoming increasingly available in stores around the country; the cabbage's ruffly leaves supply vitamin C, potassium, and lots of fiber.

1 head Napa or Chinese cabbage
1 bunch radishes, thinly sliced
2 cups fresh bean sprouts (about 1/2 pound)
1 can (8 oz.) water chestnuts, drained and sliced
2 green onions, thinly sliced
1/2 cup fresh snow peas
1/2 cup wild rice, cooked
1/3 cup vinegar (preferably white wine vinegar)
1/4 cup vegetable oil

2 tablespoons sesame oil
2 tablespoons reduced-sodium soy sauce
1 clove garlic, crushed
1/2 teaspoon ground ginger
1/2 teaspoon dried mustard

Remove five or six outer leaves from the head of cabbage, and line a large salad bowl with these leaves.

Shred remaining cabbage and place it in a second large bowl. Add radishes, bean sprouts, water chestnuts, green onions, snow peas, and wild rice.

In a small bowl, combine oils, vinegar, soy sauce, garlic, ginger, and mustard.

Pour dressing over vegetable mixture and toss. Spoon vegetable mixture into cabbage-lined salad bowl and serve.

Snappy Pea Salad
Yield: 2 servings

We love foods with plenty of crunch and color, so this salad is one of our favorite edibles. Especially appealing as a light supper, this veggie combo is a snap to assemble.

1 small head Boston or Bibb lettuce, torn into bite-size pieces
1/2 cup shelled, raw fresh peas or sliced snow peas
1 can (4 oz.) water chestnuts, drained and sliced
3 radishes, grated
1/4 cup cubed jécama
1/4 cup cubed Monterey jack cheese (optional)
2 tablespoons oil
2 tablespoons vinegar
1 tablespoon prepared mustard
1 clove garlic, crushed
1/4 cup soy baco-bits
handful alfalfa sprouts

In a large salad bowl, combine lettuce, peas, water chestnuts, radishes, jécama, and cheese. Cover and refrigerate until chilled through.

Whisk oil, vinegar, mustard, and garlic together.

Pour dressing over chilled salad; toss lightly.

Top with soy baco-bits and alfalfa sprouts.

Stimulating Springtime Salad
Yield: 6-8 servings

What a wonderful way to welcome warm weather! Fresh, supple asparagus spears, those springtime delicacies, are simply bursting with vitamins A and C as well as thiamine and riboflavin—nutrients your body needs for healthy growth and digestion.

2 pounds fresh asparagus spears
3/4 cup vegetable oil
1/3 cup tarragon vinegar
2 tablespoons sweet pickle relish
1 tablespoon chopped pimiento
1 tablespoon chopped fresh parsley
1/4 teaspoon ground black pepper
1 head Boston or Bibb lettuce, if desired
2 hard-boiled eggs, chopped (optional)

Cut off and discard about two inches on the tough end of each asparagus spear.

Steam or boil asparagus spears for 12-15 minutes or just until tender; drain and cool.

In a small bowl, combine oil, vinegar, relish, pimiento, parsley, and pepper.

Place cooked asparagus spears in a shallow bowl or dish. Pour dressing over asparagus.

Cover bowl and refrigerate asparagus for at least two hours or overnight.

To serve, drain asparagus. Arrange lettuce leaves in a large salad bowl or on individual salad plates. Arrange spears on lettuce leaves, and sprinkle egg on top.

El Cielo Salad
Yield: 4-6 servings

We call this recipe El Cielo, which is Spanish for "The Sky" and the name of a road high above our city, because this brightly colored salad makes us think of the warm days and blue skies that characterize our home. Low-calorie water chestnuts and protein-rich mung bean sprouts complement the other interesting textures in this refreshing veggie mixture.

4 cups torn romaine or other type of lettuce
4 cups torn fresh spinach
1 apple, cut into bite-size pieces
1 small red onion, sliced and separated into rings
1 cup sliced fresh mushrooms
1 can (8 oz.) sliced water chestnuts, drained
1 cup white mung bean sprouts
1/2 cup chopped tomatoes
1/2 cup Cool & Creamy Italian Dressing

Place all the ingredients, except the dressing, in a large salad bowl. Chill until serving time.

Toss with dressing.

Irwin's Waldorf Salad
Yield: 4 servings

You can certainly sink your teeth into this healthy version of everyone's favorite cool-weather salad, which generously supplies your innards with high-quality dietary fiber.

1 cup diced apples
1 cup diced celery
1/2 cup diced jécama
1/3 cup raisins
1/3 chopped walnuts
1/2 cup plain nonfat or low-fat
  yogurt (or use vanilla and/or   strawberry)
2 tablespoons mayonnaise (optional)
lettuce leaves

In a medium-sized bowl, combine apples, celery, jécama, raisins, and walnuts. Blend in yogurt.

Arrange lettuce on a serving dish or on individual salad plates, and mound salad mixture on lettuce leaves. Serve.

El Encanto Rice Salad
Yield: 4-6 servings

This unusual, fiber-rich combination of appetizing ingredients will please the most discriminating palates. A native American grain, wild rice is a nutritious delicacy that furnishes protein and B vitamins. When mixed with the sunflower seeds and yogurt in this recipe, the wild rice will help meet your body's daily protein requirements.

2 cups cooked wild rice
2 stalks celery, chopped
2 green onions, chopped
1 carrot, chopped
1 cup chopped cauliflower
1/2 cup shelled, dry-roasted sunflower seeds
1/2 cup chopped red bell pepper
1/2 cup dried apricots, diced (optional)
1/2 cup plain nonfat or low-fat yogurt
2 tablespoons Cool & Creamy Italian Dressing

In a medium-sized bowl, combine all ingredients. Chill until serving time.

Zesty Bleu Cheese Dressing
Yield: 1-1/2 cups

An aged, semi-soft cheese with lots of zip, bleu cheese complements salad greens beautifully. A bluish- green Penicillium mold endows bleu cheese with its characteristic color and pungent flavor.

1/2 cup plain nonfat or low-fat yogurt
1/2 cup mayonnaise (use commercial,
  reduced-calorie mayonnaise if   desired)
1/4 cup buttermilk
3 tablespoons crumbled bleu cheese
1 teaspoon onion powder
1/4 teaspoon garlic powder

Place all ingredients in a blender or food processor and whirl. Chill.

Cool & Creamy Italian Dressing
Yield: 2 cups

Herbs and garlic add character to this smooth, deceptively rich-tasting dressing.

1/4 cup water
1/4 cup apple cider vinegar
1 large clove garlic, minced
1 teaspoon onion powder
1 teaspoon dried savory leaves
1 teaspoon dried tarragon leaves
1 teaspoon dried basil leaves
1/2 teaspoon celery seed
1/2 teaspoon freshly ground black pepper
1/8 teaspoon dry mustard
1/2 cup safflower oil
1/2 cup olive oil

Place all the ingredients except the oil in a blender or food processor. As you whirl the ingredients together, slowly add the oil. Chill.

Lori's Green Goddess Dressing
Yield: 1-1/2 cups

Traditionally, green Goddess Dressing contains salty sardines. Here's a vegetarian, low-sodium version of the verdant blend.

1/2 cup plain nonfat or low-fat yogurt
1/2 cup mayonnaise, preferably cold-pressed
and sugar-free 1/4 cup   coarsely chopped fresh parsley
1/4 cup chopped green onions
1 clove garlic, minced
2 teaspoons lemon juice

1 teaspoon dried tarragon leaves
dash dried dill

In a jar or small bowl, mix ingredients well. Chill.

Refreshing Lemon-Cucumber Dressing
Yield: 1 quart

This dressing makes a great salad-topper for those who need to watch their fat intake—and for those who like the tang of fresh lemons. The sunflower seeds add a little extra crunch to your salad, too.

3 large cucumbers, peeled and coarsely chopped
1 cup fresh lemon juice
3/4 cup shelled, dry-roasted sunflower seeds
1/2 cup sesame oil
3 tablespoons honey
4 teaspoons tamari
1 teaspoon dried dill
1/2 teaspoon dried oregano
1/2 teaspoon garlic powder

Place ingredients in a blender or food processor and blend well. Chill.

Uplifting Lemon-Ginger Dressing
Yield: 3/4 cup

Add a taste of the Orient to you salad greens. The fresh ginger in this dressing packs a hot but slightly sweet punch.

1/2 cup sesame oil
3 tablespoons lemon juice
1 tablespoon honey
1 tablespoon minced fresh ginger
1 clove garlic, minced
1/4 teaspoon ground black pepper
dash nutmeg

Place all ingredients in a blender or food processor, and blend for at least 30 seconds. Chill.

Luscious Green Dressing
Yield: 2 cups

Breath-freshening parsley makes this refreshing dressing green and wholesome; parsley will contribute additional quantities of potassium, iron, and vitamins A and C to your already nutritious salad.

1 cup safflower or sesame oil
1 cup chopped fresh parsley (stems removed)
1/2 cup apple-cider vinegar
1/4 cup honey
1/2 ripe avocado, peeled (optional)
1 small green onion, chopped
1 teaspoon ground ginger
1/4 teaspoon (or more) curry powder
1/4 teaspoon dry mustard
1/4 teaspoon vanilla extract
1/8 teaspoon dry mustard
pinch ground black pepper

Whirl all ingredients in a food processor or blender. Chill.

Piña Colada Dressing
Yield: 2 cups

This smooth, seasoned blend contributes just the right tanginess to fresh fruit or tossed green salads.

2 cups plain nonfat or low-fat yogurt
1/2 cup unsweetened pineapple juice
1 tablespoon tamari (optional)
3/4 teaspoon garlic powder
3/4 teaspoon dried dill
1/2 teaspoon onion powder
1/2 teaspoon cumin

1/4 teaspoon paprika
dash nutmeg
1/4 cup shredded unsweetened coconut (optional)

In a small bowl or jar, mix the ingredients well. Chill.

Poppy-Seed Dressing
Yield: 2-1/2 cups

This sweet dressing tastes terrific on fresh spinach or any kind of salad greens. Use it to convert those who usually shun salads into salad enthusiasts.

1 cup safflower oil
1/2 cup water
1/2 cup honey
1/4 cup apple-cider vinegar
1/2 bell pepper, diced
3 tablespoons chopped onions
2 tablespoons prepared mustard
1 tablespoon poppy seeds
1 teaspoon dried thyme
1 teaspoon tamari (optional)

In a small bowl or jar, blend all ingredients. Chill.

Variation: Add 1/4 cup diced fresh papaya to dressing.

Hope Ranch Dressing
Yield: 2 cups

Because Hope Ranch is such a lovely Santa Barbara neighborhood, we've borrowed its name for our favorite ranch dressing, which should appeal to most salad eaters.

1 cup buttermilk
1/2 cup mayonnaise
1/2 cup plain nonfat or low-fat yogurt
1 tablespoon plus 1 teaspoon chopped fresh chives

or finely chopped green onion (tops only)
2 teaspoons chopped fresh parsley
1/4 teaspoon (or more) garlic powder
1/4 teaspoon ground cumin
1/4 teaspoon (or more) onion powder
small pinch cayenne pepper
dash paprika

In a jar or small bowl, combine all ingredients. Chill for at least one hour to allow flavors to blend.

Sass Splash
Yield: 2 cups

Like most well-balanced Italian dressings, this light "splash" accentuates the natural flavors of your salad's ingredients.

3/4 cup olive oil
2/3 cup apple-cider vinegar
1/4 cup safflower oil
1 tablespoon water
1 tablespoon grated Parmesan cheese
1 clove garlic, minced
1 teaspoon minced onion
1 teaspoon lecithin granules
1/2 teaspoon dried basil leaves
1/2 teaspoon dried parsley flakes
dash cayenne pepper

In a jar or small bowl, blend all ingredients. Chill.

Tangy Tomato Dressing
Yield: 3 cups

When you're ready for a dressing without any oil, give this piquant, easy-to-make mixture a try.

2 cups tomato juice
1 cup apple-cider vinegar
2 teaspoons dried tarragon leaves
1 teaspoon dried oregano leaves
1 teaspoon honey
1/2 teaspoon dried basil leaves
1/4 teaspoon dry mustard
1/4 teaspoon garlic powder
dash black pepper

In a large jar or medium-sized bowl, mix or shake all ingredients for about half a minute. Chill.

Kicky Tomato-Garlic Dressing
Yield: 1-1/2 cups

This nippy but slightly sweet dressing is low in fat and calories but high in vitamin C.

1 cup tomato juice
4 tablespoons safflower oil
4 tablespoons apple-cider vinegar
1 tablespoon honey
2 cloves garlic, minced
1/2 teaspoon dried basil leaves
1/2 teaspoon dried thyme leaves
1/8 teaspoon freshly ground black pepper

In a jar or small bowl, mix all ingredients. Chill.

Nanya's Vegetable Stock
Yield: 2 quarts

Named for our beloved grandmother, this vegetable broth serves as the basis for many of our soups. If you wish, you can make large quantities of the stock and freeze it.

    5 medium-sized carrots, halved
    4 medium-sized tomatoes, quartered
    3 medium-sized onions, halved
    3 celery stalks with leaves, halved
    3 sprigs parsley
    1 garlic clove, minced
    2 teaspoons dried kelp
    8 cups cold water

Place all ingredients in a large stock pot. Bring stock to a boil, reduce heat to low, and cover and simmer for one hour.

Allow to cool for 30 minutes, and then strain stock through a fine sieve.

Cool completely and refrigerate.

Buellton Barley Soup
Yield: 6 servings

An excellent source of dietary fiber, barley actually lowers cholesterol levels in our blood. In this barley soup, the addition of tomatoes and carrots gives you a pleasant dose of vitamin C, and the onions and mushrooms complement the pleasing, nutty flavor of the barley.

    6 cups Nanya's Vegetable Stock
    1/4 cup uncooked, hulled whole barley, rinsed
    1 cup sliced carrots
    1 cup fresh peas

1/2 cup sliced mushrooms
1/2 cup diced celery
1/4 cup chopped onions
1 tablespoon tamari
fresh parsley sprigs

Place stock and barley in a heavy kettle; cover and simmer until barley is tender, about one hour.

Add remaining ingredients, except the parsley, and simmer, covered, until the vegetables are barely tender.

Remove soup from heat and add the parsley. Serve.

Energizing Black-Bean Soup
Yield: 6-8 servings

Loaded with complex carbohydrates, protein, fiber, B vitamins and iron, black beans (or any kind of dry bean) give your body energy gradually. The brewer's yeast contributes additional B vitamins, protein, and minerals.

3 tablespoons olive oil
1 onion, finely chopped
1 stalk celery with leaves, chopped
6 cups Nanya's Vegetable Stock
1-1/2 cups dried black beans, picked over and rinsed
3 tablespoons brewer's yeast
2 tablespoons whole-wheat flour
1 tablespoon celery seeds
1 tablespoon tamari
freshly ground black pepper, to taste
1/2 cup fresh lemon juice
    lemon slices
1 hard-boiled egg, chopped

Heat the oil in a heavy kettle, and sauté the onion and celery in the oil until the vegetables are tender.

Add stock and beans. Bring the mixture to a boil, and then cover and simmer for three hours or until beans are tender.

Add the brewer's yeast, flour, celery seeds, and tamari.

Purée soup in batches in a food processor or blender.

Return puréed soup to the kettle and reheat, stirring, until mixture thickens slightly. Stir in the lemon juice, and add more stock or water if you find the consistency too thick.

Serve in bowls, and top each serving with lemon slices and chopped egg.

Our Best Borscht
Yield: 6-8 servings

A Russian potage, borscht is a wonderfully satisfying, naturally sweet soup made from crimson-colored beets. Serve it with a crusty, whole-grain bread, and this gratifying meal will stock your body with a variety of vitamins and minerals.

2 tablespoons oil
3 large onions, chopped
3 beets, peeled and chopped
2 beets, peeled and cubed
2 potatoes, peeled and cubed
1 medium-sized head red cabbage, shredded
1 carrot, chopped
2 quarts Nanya's Vegetable Stock
2 cups skinned, chopped fresh or canned tomatoes
2 bay leaves, crumbled
3 tablespoons brewer's yeast
1 tablespoon whole-wheat flour
1 tablespoon tamari
1/2 teaspoon freshly ground dill seeds
sour cream or yogurt

Heat the oil in a large kettle and add the onions, beets, potatoes, cabbage and carrot. Sauté for about 15 minutes.

Add vegetable stock; cover and simmer until vegetables are tender but still slightly crisp.

In a small bowl, combine tomatoes, bay leaves, brewer's yeast, whole-wheat flour, tamari, and dill seeds. Add mixture to kettle, and simmer soup for 10 minutes.

Serve in individual bowls, and top with dollops of sour cream, yogurt, or our Mock Sour Cream.

Hearty Broccoli-Cheese Soup
Yield: 6 servings

As we have said elsewhere in this book, broccoli is a nutritious vegetable with cancer-preventing properties and marvelous flavor. This recipe's combination of broccoli, cheese, and potatoes sustains your body with complete protein as well as calcium and a wide range of vitamins and minerals.

1 small bunch broccoli
1 tablespoon lemon juice
1 tablespoon safflower oil
3/4 cup chopped onion
1 clove garlic, minced
3 cups Nanya's Vegetable Stock
2 cups diced russet potatoes
1/4 teaspoon ground nutmeg
1/4 teaspoon garlic powder
1 cup low-fat milk
4 ounces cheddar cheese, shredded

Cut off broccoli flowerets, to make about 1-1/2 cups. Dice broccoli stems, to make about 1-1/2 cups.

In a small saucepan, cook flowerets in water and lemon juice until tender but still somewhat crisp. Leave flowerets in their liquid and set aside.

In a large saucepan, heat oil and add onions and garlic. Sauté until translucent and soft.

Add diced broccoli, vegetable stock, potatoes, and seasonings. Bring to a boil. Lower heat, cover, and simmer for about 50 minutes.

Transfer soup in batches to food processor or blender, and blend until smooth.

Return soup to pan and add milk, cheese, and broccoli flowerets with their liquid. Reheat soup and serve.

Sabado Tarde Celery Chowder
Yield: 6-8 servings

High-fiber celery becomes the tender, slightly crispy focus of this "Sabado Tarde" ("Saturday Afternoon") soup. Named for a street near the University of California, Santa Barbara, the soup makes us think of wintertime Saturday afternoons when we feel like eating something warm and comforting but don't want to spend much time in the kitchen.

2 cups water
4 cups chopped celery, preferably the outer
  stalks with their   leaves
1 large potato, grated
2 tablespoons butter
1 tablespoon unbleached flour
1 quart low-fat milk, scalded
1/8 teaspoon ground nutmeg
2 hard-boiled eggs, chopped
1 tablespoon tamari

Pour water into a large soup kettle and bring to a boil.

Drop the chopped celery and grated potato into the boiling water. Simmer until the celery is tender but still slightly crisp.

Meanwhile, combine the butter and flour in a medium-sized saucepan over medium heat. Gradually beat in the milk. Bring mixture to a boil and stir until it thickens slightly. Add nutmeg and stir milk mixture into the celery and potatoes in the soup kettle.

Add the eggs and tamari, and taste the soup to see whether it needs additional seasoning.

Simmer the soup, stirring continuously, until it is smooth and slightly thickened. Serve immediately.

Sunset Soup
Yield: 6-8 servings

This invigorating orange brew tastes so terrific you'll think that it's far more fattening than it is. Paradoxically, low-calorie carrots have more sugar than any other vegetable except the beet. It's no wonder that carrots lend wonderful sweetness to practically any dish they grace.

    2 tablespoons safflower oil
    1 cup chopped onions
    1-1/4 pounds finely chopped carrots
    1/4 cup finely chopped celery
    4 cups Nanya's Vegetable Stock
    1 tablespoon chopped fresh parsley
    1 bay leaf
    1/4 teaspoon dried tarragon
    3 tablespoons fresh lemon juice
    2 tablespoons tamari
    dash cayenne pepper
    sour cream or grated carrot, as desired

Heat the oil in a large saucepan. Add the onions and cook until they are light gold in color.

Add carrots, celery, stock, parsley, bay leaf, and tarragon.

Bring to a boil, lower heat, cover, and simmer for 30 minutes, or until vegetables are tender. Remove bay leaf.

Purée mixture in batches in a food processor or blender. Return soup to saucepan and bring to a boil.

Add lemon juice, tamari, and cayenne.

Serve in individual soup bowls, and garnish with dollops of sour cream or sprinklings of freshly grated carrot.

East-side Cauliflower Soup
Yield: 6 servings

A nourishing blend of cauliflower and milk, this ivory-colored potage furnishes lots of folic acid, the nutrient necessary for producing red blood cells and preventing anemia.

    1 medium-sized head cauliflower, broken into
      flowerets and steamed   until tender
    3 tablespoons butter
    2 slices onion
    1 clove garlic, minced
    1 quart milk
    2 cups low-fat milk, scalded

1 teaspoon dried kelp
1 egg yolk, lightly beaten
2 tablespoons grated Swiss or Gruyére cheese
1 vegetable bouillon cube
1 carrot, grated

Place the steamed, drained cauliflower in a food mill, food processor, or blender, and blend until smooth.

Heat the butter in a large saucepan and add the onion and garlic. Sauté until tender.

Stir the water and milk into the puréed cauliflower and add to the onion mixture. Add the dried kelp and cook for five minutes; strain.

Add a little of the hot soup to the egg yolk, and then mix the yolk into the soup in the saucepan.

Stir in the cheese and the vegetable bouillon cube. Simmer until cheese has melted and bouillon is dissolved. Serve garnished with grated carrot.

Robust Cheese Soup
Yield: 8 servings

A heartwarming blend of golden ingredients, this soup is a good source of calcium and vitamins.

1/4 pound butter or margarine
1/2 cup finely chopped carrot
1/2 cup finely chopped onion
1/2 cup finely chopped celery
1/3 cup whole-wheat pastry flour
4 cups Nanya's Vegetable Stock
3 cups (about 12 oz.) shredded cheddar cheese
1 tablespoon tamari
1 teaspoon Worcestershire sauce
1/2 teaspoon Dijon-style mustard
1/2 cup soy baco-bits

In a large saucepan, melt butter or margarine and add carrots, onion, and celery. Sauté until soft but not brown, about 15 to 20 minutes. Add flour; cook and stir mixture for about two minutes or until blended. Stir in 3 cups of stock until broth looks slightly thickened.

Transfer mixture to a blender or food processor and blend until smooth.

Place vegetable mixture to a large, clean saucepan. Stir in remaining one cup stock and the milk. Add cheese, tamari, Worcestershire sauce, and mustard. Simmer over low heat until soup is hot and cheese is melted.

Garnish each serving with soy baco-bits.

Note: This soup may be refrigerated for up to two days, or it may be frozen. Reheat slowly and do not boil.

Chumash Corn Soup
Yield: 6 servings

Named for a tribe of Indians who lived in our area not long ago, this golden soup makes a light but satisfying supper that partially meets our bodies' requirements for vitamin A. Try to use only the freshest corn; as soon as growers harvests their cobs, the natural sugars in the kernels begin to convert to starch, and the corn becomes increasingly mealy. Even in soup, corn readily reveals its age—and its sweetness!

3 cups Nanya's Vegetable Stock
1 cup fresh corn kernels
1/4 cup chopped green onions
1/2 teaspoon minced garlic
1/2 teaspoon onion powder
1/8 teaspoon dried mustard
2 cups nonfat or low-fat milk
2 ounces cheddar cheese, shredded
1 tablespoon tamari
chopped parsley for garnish

In a large saucepan, combine stock, corn, green onions, garlic, and seasonings. Bring to a boil, lower the heat, cover, and simmer for about 25 minutes.

Add milk, and simmer for five minutes longer.

Remove the corn from the soup (use a slotted ladle or a colander), and set it aside.

Pour the soup into a blender or food processor and whirl until smooth.

Return soup to saucepan; add cheese, corn, and tamari. Heat, stirring frequently, until the cheese has melted, about 5 to 10 minutes.

Serve garnished with chopped parsley.

French Basil Soup
Yield: 6-8 servings

A traditional soup from the south of France, this celebration of fresh vegetables and basil will assuredly become one of your favorite repasts. Accompanied by crusty sourdough or whole-grain bread, the soup makes fine fare for company and supplies diners with complete protein.

3 quarts Nanya's Vegetable Stock
2 cups chopped carrots
2 cups chopped white onions
1 cup diced potatoes
2 cups fresh green beans, chopped
1 cup uncooked macaroni or other small pasta
1/2 teaspoon dried kelp
1/4 cup tomato sauce
1/3 cup freshly grated Parmesan cheese
3 cloves garlic, minced
3 tablespoon finely chopped fresh basil or
  tablespoons dried basil leaves
1 tablespoon olive oil
1can (16 oz.) white beans, drained (kidney beans
  are an acceptable substitute)

Begin heating stock in a large soup kettle, and add the carrots, onions, and potatoes. Boil until they are tender but still slightly crisp.

Add the green beans, macaroni, and kelp. Simmer until the beans and macaroni are tender.

In a small bowl, combine tomato sauce, Parmesan cheese, garlic, and basil. Add the oil in a slow stream, beating vigorously.

Pour the tomato sauce mixture into the soup kettle and mix

well. Add the white beans and simmer only until beans are heated through.

Serve.

Great Galloping Gazpacho
Yield: 4-6 servings

This cold, low-sodium soup will tantalize your taste buds. Chock-full of vitamin C, it's one of the fastest, tangiest soups you can make.

2 cans (16 oz. each) unsalted tomato juice
1/4 cup wine vinegar
2 tablespoons lemon juice
2 tomatoes, diced
1 small avocado, peeled and sliced (optional)
12 ripe olives, cut into wedges
1/2 cup thinly sliced and chopped cucumber
4 green onions, including tops, chopped
1/2 teaspoon garlic powder
dash cayenne pepper
2 limes, cut into wedges

Combine tomato juice, vinegar, and lemon juice. Add vegetables and seasonings and mix well.

Chill several hours or overnight. Serve garnished with lime wedges.

Leek Soup On-the-Double
Yield: 6 servings

A simple soup to concoct, this richly flavored leek-and-potato blend supplies dietary fiber and essential nutrients like iron, niacin, and vitamin C. While the soup simmers, toss a green salad to round out your meal.

4 leeks
2 tablespoons butter or margarine

4 cups potatoes, peeled and chopped
1/2 cup diced carrots
5 cups water
1 cup nonfat or low-fat milk
1/2 teaspoon dried kelp
1/4 teaspoon freshly ground black pepper

Wash the leeks thoroughly and slice them into thin rounds. Use both the white and green parts of the leeks.

Melt the butter or margarine in a large kettle or stock pot. Add sliced leeks; cook for five minutes over medium heat or until leeks are limp.

Add potatoes, carrots, and water, and bring to a boil. Boil uncovered for 30 minutes or until potatoes are thoroughly cooked.

Add the milk, kelp, and pepper.

The soup should be thick and creamy. If you would like a smooth soup, whirl the mixture in a blender or food processor. Serve hot.

Lentil Soup De la Vina
Yield: 10 servings

Simple legumes to prepare, lentils require no soaking before you cook them, and they furnish protein, iron, B vitamins, plus the nutrients we need for strong bones—calcium and phosphorus.

1-1/2 tablespoons oil
1-1/2 cup chopped onions
1 zucchini, shredded
2 cups dried lentils, picked over and rinsed
2 quarts (approximately) cold water
2 small potatoes, scrubbed and boiled until tender
1 large carrot, grated
2 cups fresh or canned tomato juice
3/4 cup shredded cabbage
1 tablespoon tamari
10 sprigs fresh basil
1 cup shredded Monterey jack cheese
  or grated hard goat's cheese

Heat the oil in a heavy kettle or stock pot. (However, do not use an iron pot or your lentils will turn black!) Add the onions and zucchini and sauté until they are translucent.

Add the lentils and water. Bring mixture to a boil, and simmer over low heat until the lentils are tender, about one hour. Watch the water level in the pot, and add water as necessary to keep the lentils covered.

Peel and dice potatoes; add to lentil mixture.

Add carrot, cabbage, tomato juice, and tamari. Return soup to a boil, and cook until cabbage wilts.

Garnish with basil sprigs, and serve with Monterey jack or goat's cheese.

West Coast Minestrone
Yield: 8-10 servings

Everyone's favorite soup, minestrone is loaded with vitamin C and dietary fiber. Low in sodium, our version of the classic vegetable union is seasoned subtly with garlic and herbs.

1 quart water
2 medium carrots, cut into small cubes
1./2 small head of cabbage, shredded
1 medium potato, diced
1 can (16 oz.) unsalted tomatoes
1 vegetable bouillon cube
2 tablespoons olive oil
1 medium onion, sliced
2 stalks celery, sliced diagonally
1 zucchini, sliced
2 cloves garlic, minced
1 teaspoon dried kelp
1/2 teaspoon dried basil leaves
1/2 teaspoon dried marjoram leaves
1/8 teaspoon freshly ground pepper
1 cup cooked navy beans
1 can (8 oz.) unsalted tomato sauce (optional)
2 tablespoons chopped fresh parsley

Pour water into a 6-8 quart kettle or stock pot. Add carrots, cabbage, potato, tomatoes, and bouillon cube. Bring to a boil, reduce heat, and simmer for about three minutes.

In a large skillet, sauté onions in oil until translucent. Add celery, zucchini, garlic, kelp, basil, marjoram, and pepper. Continue to sauté until vegetables are tender. Add onion mixture to soup kettle.

Add beans, tomato sauce, and parsely to the soup, and simmer uncovered for 20 minutes. Add more water if the soup becomes too thick.

Serve hot.

Samarkand Soybean Soup
Yield: 4-6 servings

If you are looking for the ultimate entrée soup, this is it. This recipe's combination of soybeans, barley, bulgur, peas, and lentils offers exceptional complete protein that will restock your body's energy reserves.

1 cup dried soybeans, picked over and rinsed
1 cup whole barley, rinsed
3/4 cup bulgur (cracked wheat)
1 onion, chopped
1 clove garlic, peeled
1 teaspoon dried kelp
1 bay leaf
1 cup (total) split peas and lentils, mixed together
1 stalk celery, chopped
1/2 bell pepper, chopped
2 cups shredded kale
tamari, to taste

Place soybeans, barley, and bulgur in a large bowl. Cover mixture well with cold water, and let soak several hours or overnight.

Transfer the soybean mixture and the soaking liquid to a large kettle. Add water to a depth of two inches above the mixture. Add onion, garlic, kelp, and bay leaf. Bring to a boil, cover partly (with lid ajar), and simmer until soybeans are tender, about two hours.

Add split peas and lentils along with celery and bell pepper; continue to cook until lentils are tender. Add more water as needed.

Stir in the kale and tamari, and simmer until the kale has wilted.

Serve.

Pea Soup Lickety-Split
Yield: 6-8 servings

Although it requires a couple of hours to simmer, this thick soup is a breeze to make. Like other legumes, split peas are incredibly inexpensive, and they fortify your body with B vitamins, iron, and protein, especially when you eat them with a grain product, like bread. At meal time, you can ladle individual servings into oven-proof bowls, top them with shredded cheese, and run the bowls under the broiler.

2-1/2 cups cold water
2 cups split peas, picked over and washed
2 stalks celery with leaves, coarsely chopped
1 onion, sliced
1 large carrot, chopped
1/2 white turnip, sliced
1 bay leaf
2 tablespoons tamari
1/2 teaspoon dried savory leaves
1/4 teaspoon dried chervil

Place all the ingredients in a large kettle. Bring to a boil, reduce heat, cover, and simmer for one and one-half to two hours or until the split peas are tender.

Whirl soup in a food processor or blender until smooth.

Reheat and check seasonings.

Serve hot.

Green Spring Soup
Yield: 4-6 servings

Shallots impart delicate flavor to this perky, pea-packed soup, which proffers complete protein as well as vitamin A, potassium, iron, calcium, and phosphorus, a mineral essential to maintaining high energy levels.

1 pound tender young peas
1/2 cup water
2 tablespoons butter
1/2 cup chopped shallots or leeks (white part only)
1 small head oak-leaf, Bibb, or Boston lettuce,
 washed and drained
3 cups low-fat milk, scalded
3 vegetable bouillon cubes
1/2 teaspoon no-sodium herb-and-spice blend
1/2 teaspoon white pepper
1 cup low-fat milk

Shell the peas and place them in a large saucepan with the water. Cook the peas gently until they are barely tender. Purée in a blender or food processor and return them to the pan.

Heat the butter in a skillet and sauté the shallots or leeks until they are tender. Add to pea purée.

Place lettuce and milk in a blender or food processor and process until smooth. Add to pea purée.

Season the pea mixture with bouillon cubes, vegetable salt, and white pepper. Add milk, and heat just to serving temperature. Do not boil.

Serve hot.

Stimulating Sweet Potato Soup
Yield: 8 servings

A delectable autumn soup subtly flavored with leeks and seeds, this mildly sweet concoction provides megadoses of vitamins A and C.

4 cups peeled sweet potatoes that have been cut into chunks

3 cups thickly sliced leeks or onions
3 carrots, cut into chunks
3 stalks celery, sliced into large chunks
2 quarts water
freshly ground black pepper, to taste
1/2 cup raisins
1/4 cup low-fat or nonfat milk
2 tablespoons toasted sesame seeds
1 tablespoon caraway seeds
1 tablespoon butter

Place the sweet potatoes, leeks, carrots, celery, water, and pepper in a large kettle. Bring to a boil, cover, and simmer for about 40 minutes. The soup will be lumpy.

With a slotted spoon, remove about half the carrots and celery as well as some of the firmer potato chunks. Reserve.

Purée the remaining soup in a blender, food processor, or food mill. Return the soup to the kettle and add the reserved vegetables plus the raisins, milk, sesame seeds, caraway seeds, and butter.

Reheat to serving temperature and check the seasonings. Serve.

Yanonali Yogurt-Potato Soup
Yield: 4 servings

Looking for a little protein power to carry you through the afternoon or evening? Named for a powerful Chumash Indian chief, this combination of complex carbohydrates and dairy products is an easily digested body fuel that will provide you with energy gradually.

3 cups Nanya's Vegetable Stock
2 cups finely chopped or grated potatoes
1 medium-sized onion, chopped
1 tablespoon tamari
1 teaspoon dried kelp
1 cup plain nonfat or low-fat yogurt at room temperature
3 tablespoons Parmesan cheese
3 tablespoons chopped fresh parsley

In a large saucepan, combine stock, potatoes, onion, tamari,

Instant Applesauce
Yield: 1 serving

3 medium apples
1 tablespoon apple juice
1/2 teaspoon cinnamon
1/2 cup raisins (optional)

Core and dice apples.

Purée apples in blender, a few pieces at a time. As the apples are whirling, add the apple juice.

Place freshly made applesauce in a bowl, sprinkle with cinnamon, and add raisins, if desired. Serve.

Mock Sour Cream
Yield: 1-1/4 cups

This concoction tastes even better than commercial sour cream, and it's much less fattening than the real thing. Try it on potatoes, soups, or anything else that needs a dollop of something cool and creamy.

1 cup low-fat cottage cheese
2 tablespoons buttermilk
1 tablespoon plain nonfat or low-fat yogurt
1/2—1 teaspoon fresh lemon juice

Whirl all ingredients in food processor or blender, scraping sides often. Blend until completely smooth. Chill.

Whole-Wheat Pie Crust
Yield: for single-crust pie

Our favorite pie crust combines whole-wheat flour with a little enriched, all-purpose, white flour because a crust made with the latter is easier to handle and tastes a little lighter than one made with whole-wheat flour exclusively. However, if you'd like a denser crust, use 1-1/4 cups whole-wheat flour and omit the white flour.

> 3/4 cups whole wheat flour, sifted, or 3/4 cup whole-wheat pastry flour
> 1/2 cup enriched, all-purpose flour
> 1/2 teaspoon dried kelp (optional)
> 1/4-1/3 cup vegetable oil
> 2 tablespoons ice water

Combine flour and kelp in a bowl.

Pour the oil into the flour gradually, using a fork or pastry blender to cut the oil into the flour until the mixture forms pea-size crumbs.

Add water, and mix with hands to form a round ball.

Place the ball of dough between two pieces of waxed paper and roll to about 1/8" thickness.

Gently roll dough over rolling pin, position over pie pan, and unroll.

Trim and crimp edges.

Fill as desired.

Appendices

Appendix A

Seven-Day Light-Moderate-Light Meal
Plan for Losing Weight
(calories counts are approximate)

Although we believe that most people will not need to count calories once they switch to *Double Your Energy With Half The Effort* and begin to exercise regularly, we recognize that many folks (especially those who wish to lose weight fairly quickly) will feel comfortable with calorie estimates. For that reason, we provide the following menu suggestions and their respective calorie totals. We hope that once you read the information contained in this book and develop your ability to choose wholesome foods, you will no longer need to count calories—nor even to worry about portion size. In most cases, your appetite and your food intake will mesh smoothly and naturally.

Remember to accompany all of these menus with plenty of water for good digestion.

Day One

Breakfast	Oat Float
Lunch	Egg-Ceptional Eggplant Parmesan Green Salad with Poppy-Seed Dressing
Dinner	Anacapa Antipasto Total: 1106 calories

Day Two

Breakfast	Quick Cocoana
Lunch	Pignoli Pasta Salad
	Green salad with Cool & Creamy Italian Dressing Large apple or pear

Dinner El Encanto Rice Salad

Total: 1155 calories

Day Three

Breakfast Riviera Lift

Lunch Coyote Corn Bread
Green salad with
Potent Lemon-Ginger Dressing

Dinner Ballard Bean Salad
Optional Addition: French Basil Soup

Total: 1085 calories (without soup)

Day Four

Breakfast Summerland Sunflower Cookies served
with plain nonfat yogurt

Lunch No-Fuss Tostadas served with dollops of
guacamole

Dinner Speedy Stuffed Tomatoes
served with ten whole-wheat crackers
Optional addition: Robust Cheese Soup

Total: 1116 calories

Day Five

Breakfast Crispy Rice Spice

Lunch Protein-Packed Pocket served with
California Cool Slaw
Apple or orange

Dinner El Cielo Salad with
Zesty Bleu Cheese Dressing
or bowl of Buellton Barley Soup

Total: 1085 calories

Day Six

Breakfast
Ortega-Ridge Orange Muffin
with one teaspoon butter
one glass (6 oz.) of orange juice

Lunch
Zucchini á la Zucker
two slices of whole-wheat or sourdough
bread with one teaspoon butter
one glass (8 oz.) nonfat milk

Dinner
Skinny Spuds **or**
bowl of Pea Soup Lickety-Split

Total: 1115 calories

Day Seven

Breakfast
Sunsational Cinnamon Peaches

Lunch
Surfside Stroganoff

Dinner
Quick Cuke Salad
or bowl of Yanonali Yogurt-Potato Soup

Total: 1226 calories

Appendix B

Energy Content Of Foods
(measured in calories)

Apple, one medium (2-1/2" diam.), raw	70
Apple butter, 1 tbsp.	30
Apple juice, fresh or canned, 1 cup	120
Applesauce, unsweetened, 1/2 cup	50
Apricots, dried, 5 halves	80
Apricots, fresh, 3 medium	50
Apricot nectar, canned, 1/2 cup	60
Apricots, unsweetened, canned, 4 halves	30
Asparagus, cooked spears, 1/2 cup	25
Avocado, 1/2 (3-1/2" x 4")	185
Banana, fresh, 1 small (6")	90
Barley, dry pearl, 2 tbsp.	100
Beans, black, cooked, 1/2 cup	85
Beans, garbanzo, cooked, 1/2 cup	125
Beans, Great Northern, cooked, 1/2 cup	10
Beans, green, canned or frozen, 1/2 cup	25
Beans, green, frozen in butter sauce	65
Beans, green, frozen, with mushrooms	25
Beans, kidney, cooked, 1/2 cup	115
Beans, lima, fresh, 1/2 cup	80
Beans, pinto, cooked, 1/2 cup	115
Bean sprouts, soy, cooked, 1/2 cup	20
Beans, soybeans, cooked, 1/2 cup	115
Beans, wax, canned, 1/2 cup	20
Beet greens, cooked, 1/2 cup	30
Beets, cooked, peeled, diced or sliced, 1/2 cup	55
Biscuit, baking powder, 2" diameter	110
Blackberries, canned, in syrup, 1/2 cup	85
Blackberries, fresh, 1/2 cup	40
Blueberries, canned, in syrup, 1/2 cup	115
Blueberries, fresh, 1/2 cup	45
Blueberries, frozen, sweetened, 1/2 cup	75
Bouillon, vegetable, one cube	5
Boysenberries, frozen, sweetened, 1/2 cup	70
Bran cereal, wheat (All Bran™), 1/2 cup	95

Bran flakes, wheat, 1/2 cup	100
Bran flakes, wheat, with raisins, 1/2 cup	140
Bread, banana, one slice (3-1/2" x 3-1/2" x 3/4")	130
Bread, Boston brown, one slice (3" diameter x 1/2")	70
Bread, corn, 2" square	140
Bread, cracked wheat, enriched, one slice	60
Bread, French or Vienna, one slice (1/2" thick)	55
Bread, Italian, one slice	50
Bread, raisin, one slice	65
Bread, rye, one slice	55
Bread, white, enriched, one slice	60
Bread, whole-wheat, one slice	55
Broccoli, fresh, cooked, 3/4 cup	30
Broccoli, frozen in butter sauce, 1/2 cup	60
Brussel sprouts, cooked, 5 or 6	30
Buckwheat pancake, 4" diameter	60
Bun, cinnamon, one average	160
Bun, hot cross, one average	120
Bun, raisin, one average	180
Butter, one tbsp.	100
Buttermilk, one cup	80
Cabbage, cooked, 1/2 cup	20
Cabbage, raw, shredded, one cup	25
Cabbage, red, sweet-sour, canned, 1/2 cup	20
Cake, angel food, one slice, 1/10 of average cake	145
Cake, cheesecake, one small wedge	275
Cake, coffee, apple crumb, one slice, 2" square	175
Cake, coffee, plain	200
Cake, cupcake, iced, one medium	230
Cake, fruit, dark, one slice (3" x 2-3/4" x 1/2")	140
Cake, pineapple upside-down, one slice	450
Cake, pound, one slice (3" x 2-3/4" x 1/2")	130
Cake, strawberry shortcake, one slice	400
Cantaloupe, 5" diameter, 1/2 melon	40
Carrots, canned, 1/2 cup	30
Carrots, cooked, 1/2 cup	25
Carrots, raw, one cup	40
Catsup, tomato, one tbsp.	20
Cauliflower, cooked, 1/2 cup	15
Cauliflower, frozen, 1/2 cup	20
Cauliflower, raw, one cup	25

Celery, diced, cooked, 1/2 cup	15
Celery, diced, raw, one cup	20
Chard, Swiss, cooked, 1/2 cup	15
Cheese, bleu or Roquefort, one ounce	105
Cheese, camembert, one ounce	85
Cheese, cheddar, one ounce	115
Cheese, cottage, creamed, 1/2 cup	105
Cheese, cream, one ounce (2 tbsp.)	100
Cheese, Edam, one ounce	85
Cheese, Limburger, one ounce	100
Cheese, Parmesan, one ounce	110
Cheese spread, pimiento, one ounce	75
Cheese, Swiss, one ounce	105
Coconut, dried, shredded, 2 tbsp.	85
Coconut, fresh meat, one piece (1" x 1" x 3/4")	55
Cole slaw, with dressing, 1/2 cup	70
Collards, cooked, 1/2 cup	40
Corn, canned, 1/2 cup	70
Corn, canned, cream-style, 1/2 cup	90
Corn, fresh, one ear, 5" long	85
Corn, with carrots, pearl onions, and cream sauce, frozen, 1/2 cup	120
Corn, with peas and tomatoes, frozen, 1/2 cup	70
Corn bread muffin, one medium	130
Cornflakes, one cup	95
Cornmeal, cooked, 1/2 cup	130
Cookies, macaroon, one	105
Cookies, oatmeal, one	85
Crackers, animal, one	10
Crackers, butter thin, one	20
Crackers, cheese tidbits, 10	20
Crackers, graham, one	30
Crackers, Matzoh, one piece (8" diameter)	80
Crackers, Ry Krisp, 2	40
Crackers, Wheat Thins, one	10
Crackers, Zwieback, one	30
Cranberries, fresh, one cup	50
Cranberry juice, 1/2 cup	80
Cranberry sauce, one tbsp.	50
Cream, half-and-half, one ounce	35
Cream, sour, 2 tbsp.	60
Cream, whipping, one tbsp.	45

Cucumber, raw, 8 slices (each 1/2" thick)	15
Currants, red, fresh, 1/2 cup	55
Custard, egg, baked, 1/2 cup	205
Dandelion greens, cooked, 1/2 cup	40
Dates, dried or fresh, pitted, 3 to 4	40
Eggs, boiled or poached, one medium	75
Eggs, omelette, plain, made with one medium	120
Eggs, scrambled, made with one medium	120
Egg whites, raw, one medium	15
Egg yolks, raw, one medium	60
Eggplant, raw, 1/2 cup	25
Endive, raw, 20 long leaves	20
Escarole, 2 large leaves	10
Farina, enriched, cooked, 1/2 cup	55
Figs, canned in syrup, 3 small	135
Figs, dried, 2 small	80
Figs, fresh, 3 small	80
Figs, Kadota, 3 small	45
Gooseberries, fresh, 1/2 cup	40
Grapefruit, canned, in syrup, 1/2 cup	40
Grapefruit, fresh, 1/2 medium	80
Grapefruit juice, unsweetened, 1/2 cup	45
Grape juice, 1/2 cup	80
Grapes, Concord, 22	70
Grapes, Thompson seedless, 1/2 cup	65
Guava, fresh, one medium	70
Honey, strained, one tbsp.	65
Honeydew melon, fresh, 1/2 small (5" diameter)	30
Ice cream, chocolate, 1/2 cup	210
Ice Cream, dietetic, vanilla, 1/2 cup	175
Ice cream, strawberry, 1/2 cup	170
Ice cream, vanilla, 1/2 cup	195
Ice milk, chocolate, 1/2 cup	145
Ice milk, strawberry, 1/2 cup	135
Ice milk, vanilla, 1/2 cup	135
Ice, orange sherbet, 1/2 cup	175

Ice pop (popsicle), 4 ounces	95
Jams, marmalade, one tbsp.	55
Jellies, fruit, one tbsp.	50
Jell-O, one serving (5 per package)	65
Kale, cooked, one cup	40
Kumquats, fresh, 5 to 6 medium	65
Lemon, fresh, one medium	30
Lemonade, one cup	110
Lemon juice, 1/2 cup	30
Lentils, cooked, 1/2 cup	100
Lettuce, one small leaf	5
Lime, fresh, one large	40
Loganberries, fresh, 1/2 cup	60
Macaroni and cheese, baked, one cup	365
Macaroni, cooked, 1/2 cup	105
Macaroon, one large	105
Mango, fresh, one small	65
Maple syrup, one tbsp.	50
Margarine, one tbsp.	100
Marshmallow topping, 2 tbsp.	100
Mayonnaise, one tbsp.	100
Milk, buttermilk, 8 ounces	100
Milk, evaporated, 2 tbsp.	45
Milk, low-fat, 8 ounces	120
Milk, nonfat (skim), 8 ounces	80
Milk, whole, 8 ounces	160
Molasses, one tbsp.	50
Muffins, bran, one medium	105
Muffins, cornmeal, one medium	130
Mushrooms, canned, 1/2 cup	15
Mushrooms, fresh, 10 small	15
Muskmelon, 1/2 melon	50
Mustard greens, cooked, 1/2 cup	20
Mustard, prepared, one tbsp.	10
Nectarines, fresh, 2 medium	60
Noodles, egg, cooked, one cup	110
Nuts, almonds, 15	90

Nuts, Brazil, 4	95
Nuts, cashews, roasted, 6 to 8	90
Nuts, chestnuts, 2	30
Nuts, filberts (hazelnuts), 10 to 12	95
Nuts, macadamias, 6	110
Nuts, mixed, 8 to 12	95
Nuts, peanuts, roasted, one tbsp.	85
Nuts, pecans, 12 halves	105
Nuts, walnuts, black, 2 tbsp.	95
Oatmeal, cooked, 1/2 cup	75
Oil, vegetable, one tbsp.	100
Okra, cooked, 8 to 9 pods	30
Olives, green, pickled, 2 medium	15
Olives, ripe, canned, 2 medium	25
Onions, raw, chopped, one tbsp.	5
Onions, cooked, 1/2 cup	40
Onions, green, 6 small	25
Oranges, one medium (3" diameter)	65
Orange juice, fresh, one cup	100
Orange juice, canned or frozen, unsweetened, one cup	110
Orange sections, 1/2 cup	45
Pancakes, buttermilk, one (4" diameter)	70
Papayas, fresh, 1/2 medium	40
Parsley, fresh, chopped, one tbsp.	1
Parsnips, cooked, 1/2 cup	50
Pasta, 2 ounces dry or one cup cooked	210
Peaches, dried, cooked, unsweetened, 5 to 6 halves with juice	110
Peaches, fresh, one medium	45
Peanut butter, one tbsp.	95
Pears, fresh, one (3" x 2-1/2")	100
Peas and carrots, cooked, drained, 1/2 cup	50
Peas, edible pod, fresh, 27 pods	30
Peas, green, cooked, drained, 1/2 cup	70
Peas, green, frozen, 1/2 cup	80
Peas, split, cooked, 1/2 cup	105
Peppers, green bell, baked without stuffing, one	15
Peppers, green bell, fresh, one (3-1/2" diam.)	20
Peppers, green, canned, sweet, 3 medium	30

Persimmons, fresh, one medium	75
Pickles, bread and butter, 4 slices	20
Pickles, dill, one large	10
Pickles, sweet, chopped, one tbsp.	15
Pickles, sweet, one (2" x 1/2")	10
Pie, apple, 4" slice	375
Pie, blackberry, 4" slice	365
Pie, blueberry, 4" slice	370
Pie, cherry, 4" slice	360
Pie, coconut custard, 4" slice	310
Pie, cream, 4" slice	300
Pie, custard, 4" slice	265
Pie, lemon chiffon with crumb crust, 4" slice	210
Pie, lemon meringue, 4" slice	280
Pie, mincemeat, 4" slice	400
Pie, peach, 4" slice	405
Pie, pecan, 4" slice	480
Pie, pineapple cheese, 4" slice	270
Pie, pumpkin, 4" slice	330
Pie, raisin, 4" slice	435
Pie, rhubarb, 4" slice	430
Pie, strawberry, single crust, 4" slice	275
Pimiento, canned, one medium	10
Pineapple, fresh, diced, one cup	75
Pineapple, fresh, sliced, one slice (3-1/2" x 3/4")	45
Pineapple juice, canned or frozen, unsweetened, 1/2 cup	60
Pizza, cheese, frozen and then baked, 4" slice	245
Plums, canned, 3 medium with 2 tbsp. syrup	90
Plums, fresh, one (2" diam.)	30
Pomegranate, fresh, pulp and seeds, one medium	90
Popcorn, popped without oil, one cup	65
Popover, one average	90
Potatoes, baked, one medium (2-1/2" diam.)	100
Potatoes, boiled, one medium (2-1/2" diam.)	80
Potatoes, creamed, 1/2 cup	115
Potatoes, hash browned, 1/2 cup	240
Potatoes, mashed with milk, 1/2 cup	80
Potatoes, mashed with milk and butter, 1/2 cup	125
Potato chips, 5 (2" diam.)	55
Pretzels, three-ring, one	10
Pretzel sticks, 10 thin	10

Prunes, dried, 5 large	135
Prunes, cooked, unsweetened,	
4 medium with 2 tbsp. juice	85
Prunes, cooked with sugar,	
4 to 5 medium with 2 tbsp. juice	120
Prune juice, canned, 1/2 cup	85
Prune whip, 1/2 cup	155
Pudding, bread, with raisins, 1/2 cup	315
Pudding, lemon sponge, one serving	115
Pudding, rice with raisins, baked, 3/4 cup	250
Pudding, tapioca, minute, 1/2 cup	135
Puffed rice, one cup	50
Puffed wheat, one cup	45
Pumpkin, canned, 1/2 cup	35
Radishes, raw, 3 small (1" diam.)	5
Raisins, cooked, sweetened, 1/2 cup with juice	110
Raisins, dried, seedless, one tbsp.	30
Raisins, dried, with seeds, 1/2 cup	190
Raspberries, black, fresh, 1/2 cup	75
Raspberries, canned, in syrup, 1/2 cup	100
Raspberries, red, fresh, 1/2 cup	60
Rhubarb, raw, diced, 1/2 to one cup	15
Rhubarb, cooked, diced, sweetened, 1/2 cup	135
Rhubarb, frozen, diced, sweetened, 1/2 cup	95
Rice, brown, cooked, 1/2 cup	120
Rice, puffed, one cup	50
Rice, white, cooked, 1/2 cup	100
Roll, whole-wheat, one average	100
Rutabagas, cooked, cubed, 1/2 cup	25
Salad dressing, bleu cheese, one tbsp.	75
Salad dressing, French, one tbsp.	60
Salad dressing, mayonnaise-based, one tbsp	60
Salad dressing, Roquefort, one tbsp.	80
Salad dressing, Russian, one tbsp.	50
Salad dressing, Thousand Island, one tbsp.	100
Salad dressing, whipped cream and fruit juice	55
Sherbet, lemon, 1/2 cup	240
Sherbet, orange, 1/2 cup	225
Shredded wheat, one large biscuit	85
Soup, asparagus, cream of, canned, one cup	90

Soup, bean, canned, one cup	145
Soup, bean, homemade, 3/4 cup	195
Soup, green pea, canned, one cup	115
Soup, minestrone, canned, one cup	85
Soup, mushroom, cream of, canned one cup	150
Soup, onion, canned, one cup	50
Soup, split pea, canned, one cup	120
Soup, tomato, canned, one cup	75
Soup, tomato vegetable, canned, one cup	65
Soup, vegetable, canned, one cup	65
Soup, vegetable, cream of, canned, one cup	85
Soybeans, cooked, 3/4 cup	135
Soybean sprouts, cooked, 1/2 cup	20
Spaghetti noodles, enriched, cooked, one cup	218
Spaghetti with tomato sauce, one cup	180
Spinach, cooked, 1/2 cup	25
Spinach, fresh, 1/2 cup	20
Spinach, frozen, 4 ounces	25
Spinach, frozen, in butter sauce, 1/2 cup	50
Squash, crookneck, cooked, 1/2 cup	20
Squash, summer, cooked, 1/2 cup	15
Squash, winter, baked, 1/2 cup	50
Squash, winter, boiled and mashed, 1/2 cup	40
Starch, pure, one tablespoon	30
Strawberries, fresh, whole, 10 large	35
Strawberries, frozen, sliced, sweetened, 1/2 cup	140
Strawberries, frozen, whole, sweetened, 1/2 cup	115
Sweet potatoes, baked, one medium (2" x 5")	180
Sweet potatoes, boiled, one large (2-1/2" x 5")	245
Tangerines, fresh, one large or 2 small	45
Tangerine juice, unsweetened, 1/2 cup	50
Tapioca dessert, apple, 1/2 cup	115
Tapioca dessert, cream pudding, 1/2 cup	135
Tartar sauce, one tbsp.	95
Tomato catsup, one tbsp.	20
Tomatoes, canned, 1/2 cup	20
Tomatoes, fresh, one small	20
Tomatoes, stewed, 1/2 cup	25
Tomato juice, canned, 1/2 cup	25
Tomato paste, canned, 1/2 cup	80
Turnip greens, canned, 1/2 cup	15

Turnip greens, cooked, 1/2 cup	20
Turnips, white root, fresh, diced, 3/4 cup	30
Turnips, white root, cooked, diced, 3/4 cup	25
Vegetable juice cocktail, 1/2 cup	20
Vegetables, mixed, canned, 1/2 cup	30
Vinegar, apple cider, one tbsp.	2
Waffle, plain, one (5-1/2" diam.)	230
Water chestnuts, 4	20
Watercress, fresh, 10 medium sprigs	2
Watermelon balls, 1/2 cup	25
Watermelon, one slice (6" diam. x 1-1/2")	170
Wheat flakes, one cup	125
Wheat flour, one tbsp.	30
Wheat, puffed, one cup	45
Wheat, shredded, one large biscuit	85
Yams, cooked in their skins, 1/2 cup	105
Yeast, active dry, one cake	10
Yogurt, flavored, low-fat, one cup	230
Yogurt, plain, nonfat, 1/2 cup	60

Appendix C

1. Energy Expenditure During Sports and Recreational Activities

To prepare this chart, we calculated the calories that a 35-year-old male, whose heart beats from 131 to 161 times a minute, would expend while he exercised. The sports listed include both aerobic and anaerobic activities. To learn which sports qualify as aerobic—those that improve your cardiovascular system and burn fat—see Chapter Four.

Calories per hour above baseline expenditure

Badminton	400
Boxing	700
Baseball	850
Basketball	550
Boating, rowing slowly	400
Boating, rowing fast	800
Boating, motor	150
Bowling	250
Calisthenics	500
Cycling, slowly	300
Cycling, strenuously	600
Croquet	250
Dancing, slow step	350
Dancing, fast step	600
Field hockey	500
Fishing, from boat or pier	150
Football	600
Gardening, leisurely	250
Gardening, much lifting & stooping	400
Golfing	250
Handball	550
Horseback riding	250
Hunting	400
Jogging	600
Karate	600
Miscellaneous activities requiring some arm movement done while standing	150

Miscellaneous activities that are most strenuous done while sitting	150
Motorcycling	150
Motorscootering	100
Piano playing, leisurely	75
Piano playing, rapidly with much arm movement	125
Pipe organ playing, with much arm and leg movement	150
Reading	25
Running, fast pace	900
Singing	50
Shuffleboard playing	250
Skating, leisurely	400
Skating, rapidly	600
Skiing	450
Squash	550
Soccer	650
Swimming, leisurely	400
Swimming, rapidly & competitively	800
Tennis, singles	450
Tennis, doubles	350
Volleyball	350
Walking, leisurely	200
Walking, moderately to fast	300
Watching movies	25
Watching television	25
Wrestling	800

2. Energy Expenditure During Occupational and Household Activities

Calories per hour above baseline expenditure

Activity	Calories
Activities performed while sitting that require minimal arm movement	50-75
Activities performed while sitting that require vigorous arm movement	150-175
Activities performed while standing that require minimal arm movement	100-125
Activities performed while standing that require moderate arm movement	200-225
Answering telephone	50
Bathing	100-125
Bench work, sitting	75-100
Bench work, standing	125-150
Bookkeeping	50
Brushing teeth or hair	100-125
Carpentry, light work	200-225
Carpentry, heavy work	350-375
Dictating/Taking dictation	50
Dishwashing, routinely	75-100
Dishwashing, heavy items/rapid pace1	25-150
Dressing and undressing	50-75
Driving auto	50
Driving truck	100
Driving tractor	125-150
Dusting furniture	150-175
Filing	200-225
Gardening, leisurely	225-250
Gardening, fast or heavy work	375-400
Hammering	225-250
Hoeing	375-400
Housework, routinely/leisurely	100-125
Housework, spring and fall cleaning/much lifting	200-225
Ironing, small items/regular speed	100-125
Ironing, large items/strenuous speed	200-225

Knitting	50
Laundering, small items by machine	200-225
Laundering, large items by machine	250-275
Light polishing and waxing, regular speed	200-250
Light polishing and waxing, fast speed	250-300
Mopping floors, routinely	200-225
Mopping floors, vigorously and quickly	300-325
Preparing and cooking food, routinely	100-125
Preparing and cooking food, rapidly	150-175
Reading	25
Scrubbing floors, routinely	200-225
Scrubbing floors, vigorously and rapidly	300-325
Sewing	50
Sweeping floors	150-175
Typing	50
Walking up and down stairs	800-825
Writing	50

Appendix D

Buying Calendar for Fresh Produce

January

potatoes, turnips, cabbage, onions, Brussels sprouts, avocados, apples, oranges, tangerines, grapefruit, bananas

February

potatoes, cabbage, broccoli, celery, Brussels sprouts, apples, oranges, grapefruit, rhubarb

March

potatoes, broccoli, cabbage, celery, asparagus, avocados, apples, bananas, oranges, grapefruit, rhubarb

April

potatoes, cabbage, carrots, artichokes, lettuce, asparagus, green peas, avocados, bananas, oranges, grapefruit, pineapple, rhubarb, strawberries

May

potatoes, onions, lettuce, green beans, green peas, asparagus, various melons, apricots, peaches, cherries, pineapple, strawberries

June

potatoes, onions, lettuce, green beans, green peas, beets, sweet corn, okra, radishes, tomatoes, apricots, peaches, plums, cherries, nectarines, melons (including watermelons), blueberries, strawberries

July

cabbage, sweet corn, lettuce, green beans, beets, okra, tomatoes, lemons, peaches, plums, apricots, nectarines, melons, all kinds of berries, grapes

August

sweet corn, beets, eggplant, okra, lettuce, tomatoes, berries, melons, pears, nectarines, peaches, plums, apricots, grapes

September

beets, eggplant, okra, artichokes, lettuce, melons, grapes, apples, bananas, peaches, plums, nectarines, pears

October

cabbage, Brussels sprouts, potatoes, sweet potatoes, turnips, cauliflower, squashes, pumpkins, onions, artichokes, avocados, apples, bananas, pears, grapefruit, oranges, honeydews, grapes, cranberries

November

potatoes, sweet potatoes, turnips, cauliflower, cabbage, Brussels sprouts, onions, squashes, avocados, apples, pears, bananas, oranges, tangelos, tangerines, grapefruit, grapes, cranberries

December

potatoes, sweet potatoes, Brussels sprouts, onions, apples, bananas, pears, oranges, tangelos, tangerines, grapefruit, limes, cranberries.

A Glossary of
Key Ingredients

Avocado. A scrumptious addition to salads and sandwiches, this subtropical fruit furnishes a healthy dose of B vitamins and moderate amounts of vitamins A and C, folic acid, potassium, and protein. However, the avocado also possesses a high calorie count, and about 85 percent of those calories are fat (though monounsaturated). Therefore, we recommend enjoying "alligator pears" in moderation. The Hass and Fuerte varieties are particularly flavorful.

Basil. A plant related to mint, this mellow, slightly sweet herb plays an important role in tomato-based dishes. Fresh or dried, basil adds a taste of anise and cloves as well as a touch of Italy to salad dressings and pasta sauces.

Bran, oat. This miracle food provides protein, complex carbohydrates, and thiamin, plus its soluble fiber significantly lowers the so-called "bad" LDL (low-density lipoprotein) cholesterol in our blood. (See Chapter Two for a discussion of "good" and "bad" cholesterol.) In addition, oat bran helps to control blood sugar levels in diabetics. Recently, medical researchers found that eating 50 grams (about three muffins' worth) of oat bran drastically reduces one's serum cholesterol and helps protect against heart disease.

Bran, wheat. The outer coating of the grain's kernel, wheat bran is an excellent source of iron, phosphorus, niacin, thiamine, riboflavin, and essential fatty acids. Containing primarily insoluble fiber, wheat bran helps keep digestive tracts in good working order.

Brewer's Yeast. A non-leavening form of yeast microorganism, this food supplement adds bulk to almost any dish and is a super source of key nutrients, including protein, B vitamins, and various minerals. To improve your glucose metabolism, buy brewer's yeast as flakes or powder and sprinkle it in soups, casseroles, and batter for baked goods. (Because it tastes slightly bitter, brewer's yeast is most palatable when combined with other ingredients.)

Bulgur. A staple in Middle Eastern cuisine, bulgur is wheat that has been steamed, dried, and cracked into small granules (the darker the better). Supermarkets sell it in boxes, and health food stores generally sell it in bulk. Full of fiber, essential amino acids, vitamins, and minerals, deliciously nutty bulgur makes an appealing alternative to rice.

Butter. A highly saturated and cholesterol-laden fat made from dairy milk or cream, butter makes a delicious but potentially artery-damaging spread on baked goods and other foods. Nonetheless, when we need only small amounts of a solid fat for a recipe or a spread, we generally prefer butter to margarine because butter tastes far superior and is a completely natural product. (Margarines contain hydrogenated fat, a problem we discuss in Chapter Two.) For a real taste treat, try raw certified butter, an unprocessed, unsalted sensation.

Flaxseed. Also known as linseed, this herbal supplement has an effective, natural laxative effect. Add it to baked goods or casseroles, but be aware that flaxseed can interfere with your body's ability to absorb iron. Also, do not use the seed if your are pregnant or breast-feeding, and do not feed it to young children; flaxseed may contain naturally produced toxins that usually cause no problems for adults but which may be harmful to babies and children.

Grains. These are the seeds or fruits of cereal grasses, the food family that offers essential amino acids, vitamins, minerals, and large quantities of fiber. Grains include wheat, oats, rice, corn, millet, rye, barley, sorghum, and amaranth. When we discuss grains in our text, we're also talking about bread, pasta, pancakes, hot and cold cereals, or any other edible product that includes a grain as a main ingredient.

Honey. A completely natural sweetener, honey usually tastes sweeter per teaspoon and per calorie than table sugar, and it contains small amounts of minerals, vitamins, and amino acids. Nonetheless, its nutritive value is minimal, and it consists of more than 80 percent sugar by weight, so we call only for small amounts of honey in our recipes. We recommend *emphatically* that you do not give honey to children under one year of age, whose gastrointestinal tracts cannot deal with the botulism that may be present in honey.

Jícama. (HIC-cah-ma) Low in calories but high in flavor, this sweet-tasting tuber has a brown skin and a crisp, white flesh similar to that of a water chestnut. Although jícamas have little nutritive value, they contribute a flavorful crunch to salads or stir-fried veggie dishes. Peel jícamas before slicing them into strips or cubes.

Kale. A relative of cabbage, this curly, dark-green vegetable possesses cancer-preventing properties. Usually served cooked, kale is low in calories but rich in protein, iron, potassium, calcium, and vitamins A and C.

Kelp. The leaves of this seaweed normally come dried and serve as a tasty seasoning for soups and casseroles. Kelp also makes a good bulking agent that aids intestinal processes, and it contains the chemicals bromine, iodine, potassium and sodium. If you have an iodine sensitivity or are pregnant, consult your health care provider before sprinkling this supplement on foods.

Legumes. Extremely versatile peas and beans, the legume family includes peanuts, lentils, chickpeas (garbanzo beans), black beans, white beans, split peas, kidney beans, lima beans, pinto beans, black-eyed peas, red beans, and soybeans. These pod-grown vegetables are exceptionally high in protein, and they supply our bodies with lysine, an essential amino acid that's practically missing in grains. Combined with grains, legumes provide humans with usable, easily digested protein. These peas and beans also furnish minerals and plenty of energy-raising starch.

Mayonnaise. If consumed indiscriminately, this combination of egg, oil, vinegar or lemon juice, powdered mustard, and salt can damage your arteries. Used sparingly, mayonnaise complements many foods well. Commercial versions taste okay, but homemade tastes even better and contains no additives. If you decide to follow a recipe and make your own, you can substitute egg whites for the egg and use safflower or olive oil for the requisite vegetable oil.

Millet. The seed from an Asian grass, millet contains more protein-making essential amino acids than many other grains, and it comes pearled, puffed, as small kernels known as *whole hulled groats.*, as meal, and as flour. Millet furnishes iron, manganese, phosphorus, copper, and B vitamins, especially thiamine.

Molasses, blackstrap. This thick, liquid sweetener has far more nutritive value than table sugar, fructose, or honey, for it can contain significant amounts of iron as well as some calcium and other minerals. Potent in flavor, blackstrap molasses is a by-product of the process that creates table sugar.

"Natural" foods. This frequently used term designates unprocessed foods that come to us almost directly from their original sources and to which nothing synthetic has been added.

Oils. Polyunsaturated or monounsaturated fats (see our discussion of fats in Chapter Two), oils bind other food ingredients together, add flavor, prevent food from sticking during cooking, and play an important part in helping our bodies manufacture the fat that cushions our organs. We prefer to cook with safflower or olive oils because they number among the oils most effective in reducing serum cholesterol. However, too much fat of any kind can increase body weight and heighten your chances of developing cancer and gallstones, so we use all oils in moderation.

Organic foods. These are foods that growers have raised as naturally as possible and that have not been exposed to synthetic chemicals or fertilizers.

Pasta. The Latin word for "dough" or "paste," pasta designates a whole family of variously shaped noodles made from flour (usually wheat) and water. Pasta may also contain additional ingredients for color or flavor. You can make your own or buy it dried or fresh. An amazingly versatile complex carbohydrate, pasta fills you up without filling you with calories, plus it furnishes protein, iron, riboflavin, niacin, and lots of thiamine.

Rice. An Asian grain that has furnished protein and other nutrients to multitudes for centuries, rice serves as the basis for many of our entrées and salads. Brown rice is far superior to white rice in nutritive value and in flavor; the former possesses a nutty-tasting layer of bran that supplies fiber and vitamin E. In addition, brown rice offers more protein, potassium, and phosphorus than does any shape or style of white rice.

Sprouts. When beans, grains, or seeds germinate, they shoot up tiny plants or sprouts that contain high-quality protein, vitamins, and minerals but practically no calories. Sprouts contribute flavor and crunch to practically any dish. You can find popular alfalfa, mung bean, and soybean sprouts at grocery stores, and you can purchase sprouting seeds from health food stores and easily learn to grow your own.

Tamari. This dark, naturally fermented liquid makes an excellent seasoning that's quite similar to soy sauce or *shoyu*. Look for tamari, which usually contains both soybeans and wheat as principle ingredients, at natural food stores.

Tofu. Rich in protein and calcium, inexpensive tofu is produced from curdled soy milk and formed into moist, soft blocks that possess the texture of custard but have very little flavor. Tofu, which is low in calories and fat, can replace animal meat in many dishes, and it absorbs the flavors of the foods and seasonings with which it cooks.

Whole foods. These are foods that come to us from their natural sources completely or nearly intact and to which nothing artificial has been added. Whole foods contain all the nutrients with which Nature originally supplied them.

Yogurt. The creamy result of combining milk with a bacterial culture, this centuries-old, slightly sour-tasting food offers humans protein and lots of calcium. Choose low-fat or nonfat yogurt, which generally tastes as rich and smooth as yogurt made from whole milk.

Endnotes

Chapter 1

[1] Harold McGee, *On Food and Cooking* (New York: Charles Scribner's Sons, 1984), p. 528.

[2] Lauren Lissner et al., "Dietary Fat and the Regulation of Energy Intake in Human Subjects," *American Journal of Clinical Nutrition* 46: December, 1987, pp. 891-92.

[3] Frances Moore Lappé, *Diet for a Small Planet*, Tenth Anniversary Edition (New York: Ballantine Books, 1982), p. 8.

[4] Lappé, p. 8.

[5] Jane Brody, *Jane Brody's Nutrition Book* (New York: Bantam Books, 1981; rev. 1987), p. 442.

Chapter 2

[1] Food and Nutrition Board, National Research Council, 1980, *Recommended Dietary Allowances*, 9th ed. (Washington, D.C.: National Academy of Sciences), p. 43.

[2] Harold McGee, *On Food and Cooking* (New York: Charles Scribner's Sons, 1984), p. 533.

[3] Jane Brody, *Jane Brody's Nutrition Book* (New York: Bantam Books, 1981; rev. 1987), p. 34.

[4] Frances Moore Lappé, *Diet for a Small Planet*, Tenth Anniversary Edition (New York: Ballantine Books, 1982), p. 136.

[5] Jane Brody, *Jane Brody's Good Food Book* (New York: W.W. Norton & Company, 1985), p.114.

[6] Brody, *Nutrition Book*, p. 62.

[7] Ruth L. Pike and Myrtle L. Brown, *Nutrition: An Integrated Approach*, 3rd ed. (New York: John Wiley & Sons, 1984), p. 532.

[8] Brody, *Good Food Book*, p. 11.

[9] McGee, p. 530.

[10] Brody, *Nutrition Book*, p. 73.

[11] Cited in Letitia Brewster and Michael F. Jacobson, *The*

Changing American Diet (Washington, D.C.: Center for Science in the Public Interest, 1978), p. 5.

[12]McGee, p. 528.

[13] Tatu A. Miettinen, "Dietary Fiber and Lipids," *American Journal of Clinical Nutrition*, 45 (May 1987), pp. 1237-42.

Chapter 3

[1] D.S. Minors and J.M. Waterhouse, *Circadian Rhythms and the Human* (Bristol, England: John Wright & Sons, Ltd., 1981), p. xv.

[2]Jeremy Campbell, *Winston Churchill's Afternoon Nap* (London: Aurum Press Ltd., 1988; first published by Simon and Schuster, 1986), p. 13.

[3]Campbell, p. 92.

[4]Michael E. DeBakey et al., *The Living Heart Diet* (New York: Raven Press Books, 1984), p. 49.

[5]B.J. Spring et al., "Effects of Carbohydrates on Mood and Behavior," *Nutrition Reviews* 44: May 1986, p. 51.

Chapter 4

[1]Jane Brody, *Jane Brody's Nutrition Book* (New York: Bantam Books, 1981; rev. 1987), p. 297.

[2]Cited in Joseph C. Piscatella, *Choices for a Healthy Heart* (New York: Workman Publishing, 1987), p. 190.

[3]R. Biebinski, Y. Schutz, and E. Jequier, "Energy Metabolism During the Postexercise Recovery in Man," *American Journal of Clinical Nutrition*, 42 (July 1985), p. 82.

[4]Covert Bailey, *Fit or Fat?* (Boston: Houghton Mifflin Co., 1978), pp. 9-13.

[5]Alice G. March et al., "Bone Mineral Mass in Adult Lacto-ovo-Vegetarian and Omnivorous Males." *American Journal of Clinical Nutrition*, 37 (March 1983), p. 453.

[6]If you'd like to know how to stretch effectively and comfortably for your particular sport-or simply to condition your muscles at any time of day-take a look at Bob Anderson's *Stretching...for Everyday Fitness* (New York: Random House and

Shelter Publications, 1980). The drawings will guide you through many different stretches that will make you feel limber and that can alleviate tension.

Chapter 5

[1]Cited in many places, including Joseph Piscatella's *Choices for Healthy Heart* (New York, Workman Publishing, 1987), pp. 267-8.

[2]Bernie S. Siegel, *Love, Medicine & Miracles* (New York: Harper & Row, 1986), p. 4.

[3]For an outstanding discussion about the power of hope and the process of becoming a "hardy" individual, read Dr. Joan Borysenko's *Minding the Body, Mending the Mind* (Reading, MA: Addison-Wesley Publishing Co., Inc., 1987).

[4]The Roseto study is described by Laurel Robertson, Carol Flinders, and Brian Ruppenthal in their *New Laurel's Kitchen* (Berkeley, CA: Ten Speed Press, 1986), pp. 347-49.

[5]Nancy Zi, *The Art of Breathing* (New York, Bantam Books, 1986), pp. 2-8. This how-to book provides practical and extremely valuable information on the importance of good breathing techniques.

Glossary

[1]Studies by Dr. James Anderson of the University of Kentucky at Lexington cited in Robert E. Kowalski, *The 8-Week Cholesterol Cure* (New York: Harper & Row, 1987), pp. 50-53.

Bibliography

American Dietetic Association. "Position Paper on the Vegetarian Approach to Eating." *Journal of the American Dietetic Association*, 77: 61 (1980), pp. 61-69.

Anderson, Bob. *Stretching . . . for Everyday Fitness*. New York: Random House and Shelter Publications, 1980.

Anderson, John J. B., ed. *Nutrition and Vegetarianism: Proceedings of Public Health Nutrition Update, May 1981, Chapel Hill, North Carolina*. Health Sciences Consortium, 1982.

Bailey, Covert. *Fit or Fat?* Boston: Houghton Mifflin Co., 1978.

Bielinski, R., Y. Schutz, and E. J_quier. "Energy Metabolism during the Postexercise Recovery in Man." *American Journal of Clinical Nutrition*, 42 (July 1985), pp. 69-82.

Borysenko, Joan. *Minding the Body, Mending the Mind*. Reading, MA: Addison-Wesley Publishing Co., 1987.

Brewster, Letitia and Michael F. Jacobson. *The Changing American Diet*. Washington, D.C.: Center for Science in the Public Interest, 1978.

Brody, Jane. *Jane Brody's Nutriton Book*. New York: Bantam Books, 1981; rev. 1987.

— — — — —. *Jane Brody's Good Food Book*. New York: W. W. Norton & Co., 1985.

— — — — —. *The New York Times Guide to Personal Health*. New York: Avon Books, 1982.

Campbell, Jeremy. *Winston Churchill's Afternoon Nap: A Wide-Awake*

Inquiry into the Human Nature of Time. New York: Simon and Schuster, 1986; rpt. London: Aurum Press Ltd., 1988.

Charley, Helen. *Food Science.* New York: John Wiley & Sons, 1982.

Connor, Sonja L., and William E. Connor. *The New American Diet.* New York: Simon and Schuster, 1986.

DeBakey, Michael, E., et al. *The Living Heart Diet.* New York: Raven Press Books, 1984.

Dombrowski, Daniel A. *The Philosophy of Vegetarianism.* Amherst: University of Massachusetts Press, 1984.

Dwyer, Johanna. "Wonderful World of Vegetarianism." *Nutrition and Vegetarianism: Proceedings of Public Health Nutrition Update, May 1,1981, Chapel Hill, North Carolina* Health Sciences Consortium, 1982.

Food and Nutrition Board, National Research Council, 1980. *Recommended Dietary Allowances*, 9th ed. Washington D.C.: National Academy of Sciences.

Griffith, H. Winter. *Complete Guide to Vitamins, Minerals & Supplements.* Tucson: Fisher Books, 1988.

Hill, Devra Z. *Rejuvenate: The Scientific Way to Look and Feel Younger without Drugs or Surgery.* Hollywood, CA: Irwin Zucker & Daughters, Inc., 1982.

Horton, Edward S. "Introduction: An Overview of the Assessment and Regulation of Energy Balance in Humans." *The American Journal of Clinical Nutrition*, 38 (December1983), pp. 972-77.

Kamen, Betty and Si Kamen. *Kids Are What They Eat.* New York: Arco Publishing, 1983.

Kowalski, Robert E. *The 8-Week Cholesterol Cure.* New York: Harper & Row, 1987.

Lappè, Frances Moore. *Diet for a Small Planet,* Tenth Anniversary Edition. New York: Ballantine Books, 1982.

Lissner, Lauren, et al. "Dietary Fat and the Regulation of Energy Intake in Human Subjects." *American Journal of Clinical Nutrition,* 46 (December 1987), pp. 886-92.

Mann, Jim. "Complex Carbohydrates: Replacement Energy for Fat or Useful in Their Own Right?" *American Journal of Clinical Nutrition,* 45 (May 1987), pp. 1202-6.

March, Alice G., et al. Bone Mineral Mass in Adult Lacto-ovo-vegetarian and Omnivorous Males," *American Journal of Clinical Nutrition,* 37 (March 1983), pp. 453-56.

Mateljan, George. *Healthy Living Cuisine.* Montebello, CA: Health Valley Foods, 1984.

Miettinen, Tatu A. "Dietary Fiber and Lipids." *American Journal of Clinical Nutrition,* 45 (May 1987), pp. 1237-42.

Mindell, Earl. *New and Revised Vitamin Bible.* New York: Warner Books, 1979.

—————. *Unsafe at Any Meal.* New York: Warner Books, 1987.

Minors, D. S. and J. M. Waterhouse. *Circadian Rhythms and the Human.* Bristol, England: John Wright & Sons, Ltd., 1981.

Murphy, J. "Another Reason for Vegetarianism." *The Journal of the American Medical Association,* 255 (Jan. 3, 1986), pp. 666 ff.

Nomura, A., L. K. Heilbrun, and G. N. Stemmerman. "Prospective Study of Coffee Consumption and the Risk of Cancer." *Journal of the National Cancer Institute,* 76 (April 1986), pp. 587 ff.

Piscatella, Joseph C. *Choices for a Healthy Heart.* New York: Workman Publishing, 1987.

Pollitt, Ernesto and Peggy Amante, eds. *Energy Intake and Activity.* Current Topics in Nutrition and Disease, Volume 11. New York: Alan R. Liss, Inc., 1984.

Potter, J. D. and A. J. McMichael. "Diet and Cancer of the Colon and Rectum: A Case-Control Study." *Journal of the National Cancer Institute,* 76 (April 1986), pp. 557 ff.

Robertson, Laurel, Carol Flinders, and Brian Ruppenthal. *The New Laurel's Kitchen.* Berkeley, CA: Ten Speed Press, 1986.

Siegel, Bernie S. *Love, Medicine & Miracles.* New York: Harper & Row, 1986.

Silverstone, Trevor, ed. *Appetite and Food Intake: Report of the Dahlem Workshop on Appetite and Food Intake, Berlin 1975.* Berlin: Abakon Verlagsgesellschaft, 1976.

Spring, B. J. et. al. "Effects of Carbohydrates on Mood and Behavior." *Nutrition Reviews,* 44 (May 1986), pp. 51 ff.

U.S. Department of Health and Human Services, Public Health Service, National Institutes of Health. *Diet, Nutrition & Cancer Prevention: A Guide to Food Choices.* NIH Publication No. 85-2711, November 1984.

Zi, Nancy. *The Art of Breathing.* New York: Bantam Books, 1986.

Recipe Index

Sandwiches
Invigorating Tofu-Salad Sandwich 85
Protein-Packed Pocket 75
Speedy Sprice Sandwich 62

Snacks
Banana Breakfast Custard 48
Carob Fudge Balls 49
Los Padres Granola 52
Summerland Sunflower Cookies 49
Sunup Pudding 55
Surf's Up Soyuncream 54

Soups (118-133)
Buellton Barley Soup 118
Chumash Corn Soup 125
East-side Cauliflower Soup 123
Energizing Black-Bean Soup 119
French Basil Soup 126
Great Galloping Gazpacho 127
Green Spring Soup 132
Hearty Broccoli Cheese Soup 121
Leek Soup On-the-Double 127
Lentil Soup De la Vina 128
Nanya's Vegetable Stock 118
Our Best Borscht 120
Pea Soup Lickety-Split 131
Robust Cheese Soup 124
Sabado Tarde Celery Chowder 122
Samarkand Soybean Soup 130
Stimulating Sweet Potato Soup 132
Sunset Soup 122

West Coast Minestrone 129
Yanonali Yogurt-Potato Soup 133
Sour Cream, Mock 134
Stock, Nanya's Vegetable 118

Vegetable Dishes
Alamar Eggplant Medley 91
Anacapa Antipasto 61
Cabana Curried Rice 90
Calle Real "Creamed" Vegetables 68
Country-Club Asparagus 88
County Bowl Cabbage Rolls 78
Cuyama Carrots 98
Egg-ceptional Eggplant Parmesan 70
El Colegio Curried Cauliflower 69
Franceschi Stuffed Peppers 82
Garden Street Ratatouille 71
La Playa Potatoes 72
Lively, Lemony Beans 93
Mushrooms Arlington 63
Padaro Lane Potatoes 92
Palm Park Peas 96
Pizzazzy Pizza Toppings 77
Potato Crisps 97
Short-Order Sweet Potatoes 90
Sisquoc Squash 82
Skinny Spuds 94
Speedy Stuffed Tomatoes 88
Stimulating Springtime Salad 109
Tomatoes Montecito 89
Zucchini à la Zucker 85
Whole-Wheat Pie Crust 135

General Index

About the Authors:

Judi and Shari Zucker, who enjoy a well-deserved reputation as the "Double-Energy Twins," began their vegetarian life style as well as their career as cookbook writers while they were high school students and track stars. The twins learned early that nutritious, whole foods gave them sustained energy and helped them to break the women's one- and two-mile track records at Beverly Hills High School. (No one has yet beaten their records.) Enthusiastic about sharing their energy secrets, they published *How to Survive Snack Attacks . . . Naturally* in 1979, when they were just seventeen years old. The book enjoyed such success that Judi and Shari soon followed their first cookbook with *How to Eat without Meat . . . Naturally* in 1981.

The Zuckers continued their study of health and nutrition at the University of California, Santa Barbara, where they graduated with honors in Ergonomics, the study of human physiology, physical education, and nutrition.

Following graduation, Judi and Shari served as media specialists for General Mills, whose representatives had asked the twins to publicize the company's Nature Valley Granola products. After promoting and demonstrating healthy snacks on a six-week "Snack Sense" tour, the twins realized that they wanted to provide the public with additional information about sound diet and exercise programs.

Although Judi and Shari are now exceptionally successful in their respective professions, real estate and interior design, the twins continue to create and compile recipes for nutritious, low-fat, high-fiber foods. They also plan to package and market their delicious "Zookie Cookie," a delectably wholesome morsel for which they have developed a closely guarded, exclusive recipe. In addition, the Zuckers appear on national and local television talks shows, teach natural-food cooking classes for local adult education programs, and maintain their own fitness by walking, running, swimming, biking, or playing tennis every day.